Workbook for

Lippincott's Advanced Skills
for Nursing Assistants

PAMELA J. CARTER, RN, BSN, MEd, CNOR
Program Coordinator/Instructor
School of Health Professions
Davis Applied Technology College
Kaysville, Utah

AMY J. STEGEN, RN, BSN, MSN
Nursing and Allied Health Coordinator
School of Health Professions
Davis Applied Technology College
Kaysville, Utah

 Wolters Kluwer | Lippincott Williams & Wilkins
Health
Philadelphia · Baltimore · New York · London
Buenos Aires · Hong Kong · Sydney · Tokyo

Ancillary Editor: Season Evans
Production Project Manager: Cynthia Rudy
Director of Nursing Production: Helen Ewan
Senior Managing Editor / Production: Erika Kors
Design Coordinator: Holly Reid McLaughlin
Manufacturing Coordinator: Karin Duffield
Production Services / Compositor: Aptara, Inc.

9 8 7 6 5 4 3 2 1

Printed in the United States of America

ISBN: 978-0-7817-9792-4

Care has been taken to confirm the accuracy of the information presented and to describe generally accepted practices. However, the authors, editors, and publisher are not responsible for errors or omissions or for any consequences from application of the information in this book and make no warranty, expressed or implied, with respect to the currency, completeness, or accuracy of the contents of the publication. Application of this information in a particular situation remains the professional responsibility of the practitioner; the clinical treatments described and recommended may not be considered absolute and universal recommendations.

The authors, editors, and publisher have exerted every effort to ensure that drug selection and dosage set forth in this text are in accordance with the current recommendations and practice at the time of publication. However, in view of ongoing research, changes in government regulations, and the constant flow of information relating to drug therapy and drug reactions, the reader is urged to check the package insert for each drug for any change in indications and dosage and for added warnings and precautions. This is particularly important when the recommended agent is a new or infrequently employed drug.

Some drugs and medical devices presented in this publication have Food and Drug Administration (FDA) clearance for limited use in restricted research settings. It is the responsibility of the health care provider to ascertain the FDA status of each drug or device planned for use in his or her clinical practice.

Preface

Workbook for Lippincott's Advanced Skills for Nursing Assistants, developed alongside *Lippincott's Advanced Skills for Nursing Assistants* with the aid of an instructional design team, is designed to help students internalize and apply the important concepts and facts presented in the textbook. Students will benefit from first reading the assignment in the textbook and then completing the corresponding workbook assignment. This approach allows students to review and reinforce the information that they have just read. In addition, after working on the workbook assignment, students who are having difficulty understanding the information presented in the textbook will know what type of questions they need to ask in class the following day. This ability to recognize areas of difficulty helps students to better utilize instruction time.

A UNIQUE ORGANIZATION

The organization of each chapter in *Workbook for Lippincott's Advanced Skills for Nursing Assistants* follows the same organization as the corresponding chapter in *Lippincott's Advanced Skills for Nursing Assistants*. This unique organization enhances flexibility with regard to assignments—it is easy to assign all, or just part of, a workbook chapter, according to the needs of your particular curriculum. In addition, this unique organization allows students to identify particular areas of difficulty where more clarification and review are needed. **Key Learning Points,** derived from the learning objectives in the textbook, are given for each subtopic in the chapter and help the student to identify the concepts that are being reviewed and reinforced.

ACTIVITIES DESIGNED TO APPEAL TO DIFFERENT TYPES OF LEARNERS

This workbook uses several different types of activities to help students internalize and apply the information in the textbook. A wide variety of activities is important for appealing to students with different learning styles. Variety also helps to keep students engaged in the assignment. Some of the activity types that you will find in this workbook include:

- **Multiple-choice questions:** Select the single best answer from four choices.
- **Fill-in-the-blanks:** Complete a phrase or sentence.
- **Think About It!** Write a short response to a thought-provoking "what if?" scenario.
- **Matching:** Match the terms or pictures to their descriptions.
- **Labeling:** Fill in the missing labels on a key piece of artwork.
- **Sequencing:** Put the steps of a procedure or process in the correct order.
- **Identification:** Recognize the phrases or sentences that apply to a given situation.

Answers to the activities in *Workbook for Lippincott's Advanced Skills for Nursing Assistants* are provided on the Instructor's Resource DVD and on thePoint,* a Web-based course and content management system (http://thePoint.lww.com/CarterAdvancedSkills) so that they may be given to the students at the instructor's discretion.

PROCEDURE CHECK-OFF LISTS

In addition to a variety of activities designed to reinforce the information in Chapters 1 through 15 of *Lippincott's Advanced Skills for Nursing Assistants*, this workbook contains procedure check-off lists. These check-off lists are very useful during the laboratory portion of the course, when students are practicing the procedures they have just learned.

It is our sincere hope that students will find the *Workbook for Lippincott's Advanced Skills for Nursing Assistants* fun as well as educational. As always, we welcome and appreciate feedback from our readers.

Pamela J. Carter
Amy J. Stegen

*thePoint is a trademark of Wolters Kluwer Health.

Contents

CHAPTER 1

Working in an Advanced Care Setting

RESPONSIBILITIES OF THE NURSING ASSISTANT IN THE ADVANCED CARE SETTING

Key Learning Points

- Three factors that can put a person in need of advanced (acute) care
- Health care settings where advanced care may be provided
- The importance of providing holistic, humanistic care in the advanced care setting
- Changes in the health care industry that have led to changes in the way unlicensed health care workers, such as nursing assistants, are being trained and used

Activity A *Think About It! Briefly answer the following questions in the space provided.*

In an advanced (acute) care setting, acutely ill people are provided a high level of care. Today, advanced care is available in many different types of health care settings.

1. Why is advanced care now being made available in health care settings other than a hospital?

_____

_____

_____

2. What are the other health care settings that provide advanced nursing care?

_____

_____

_____

Activity B *Select the single best answer for each of the following questions.*

1. A nursing assistant was allowed to provide tracheostomy care in her previous job. However, she is not sure if she is allowed to perform that skill in her present job. What should the nursing assistant do before performing tracheostomy care in her new job?
   a. Assume that this facility allows her to do the same skills as the old job allowed.
   b. Go ahead and perform tracheostomy care because she is trained to do so and ask her supervisor when she sees her next.
   c. Check the listed tasks in her textbook.
   d. Check with her supervisor first.

2. Which of the following best describes cross-training?
   a. Teaching long-tenured employees how to improve their performance
   b. Teaching employees skills that are not usually within their scope of practice
   c. Teaching new employees skills that are within their scope of practice
   d. Teaching employees soft skills to help them in their routine work life

1

Activity C *Think About It! Briefly answer the following question in the space provided.*

A nursing supervisor has assigned a nursing assistant certain advanced skills that are part of the nursing assistant's job description. However, some of the nursing staff are still hesitant to agree that nursing assistants should be performing advanced skills. Discuss ways that the nursing assistant can earn the respect of co-workers.

_____

_____

_____

Activity D *Fill in the blanks using the words given in brackets.*

[invasive, education, nurse, unstable]

1. An acutely ill person is one who has a severe illness or whose condition is _____.

2. Nursing assistants help the _____ by performing basic nursing functions.

3. Continuing _____ involves asking questions, reading nursing journals, and taking advantage of any in-service education offered by the facility.

4. _____ tasks performed by health care workers involve inserting equipment into the patient's body or breaking the skin.

Activity E *Place an "X" next to each correct answer for the following questions.*

1. Which of the following titles may be used for a nursing assistant?
   a. _____ Phlebotomist
   b. _____ Patient care assistant
   c. _____ Licensed nurse
   d. _____ Patient care technician
   e. _____ Health care assistant

2. Which of the following factors has contributed to the changes in the way health care is delivered today?
   a. _____ Increase in cost of health care
   b. _____ Increased nursing responsibilities
   c. _____ Nursing shortage
   d. _____ Insurance plans
   e. _____ Increase in hospitals

Activity F *Fill in the blanks using the words given in brackets.*

[isolation, complex, empathy, culture, spiritual]

1. Health care workers should imagine how it would feel to be in the patient's situation and act with _____ and compassion.

2. The health care worker should not only consider the patient's physical needs but also the patient's emotional, social, and _____ needs.

3. The technology, _____ treatments, and fast-paced environment can make it difficult for the health care professional to look past the person's illness or condition.

4. _____ precautions may make the patient feel lonely.

5. Health care workers should consider the patient's _____ and age when providing care.

QUALITY CONTROL IN THE ADVANCED CARE SETTING

Key Learning Point

■ Role of the United States government and independent organizations (such as The Joint Commission) in ensuring quality patient care

Activity G *Select the single best answer for each of the following questions.*

1. In which year was The Joint Commission on Accreditation of Healthcare Organizations established?
   a. 1941
   b. 1950
   c. 1951
   d. 1959

2. What was implemented by The Joint Commission to enhance the credibility of the accreditation process?
   a. Gathering accounting records
   b. Unannounced on-site survey visits
   c. Additional legal procedures
   d. Gathering evidence through questionnaires

Activity H *Think about It! Briefly answer the following question in the space provided.*

The Joint Commission, known in the past as The Joint Commission on Accreditation of Healthcare Organizations (JCAHO), is an organization that helps to ensure that facilities provide quality health care. List two standards established by The Joint Commission that work to meet this goal.

_____

_____

_____

DELEGATION

Key Learning Points

- The five rights of delegation
- How the nurse and the nursing assistant use the five rights of delegation to ensure that the care provided is safe and legal
- The nurse's responsibilities with regard to delegation
- The nursing assistant's responsibilities with regard to delegation

Activity I *Think About It! Briefly answer the following questions in the space provided.*

1. The five rights of delegation act as guidelines for nurses to decide which tasks to delegate. They also help nursing assistants decide which delegated tasks to accept. List the five rights of delegation.

_____

_____

_____

2. The nursing team will function efficiently if the nurses and the nursing assistants perform their delegated tasks responsibly without causing harm to the patient. Nurses have the authority to delegate selected tasks to nursing assistants. List and describe two responsibilities of the nurse regarding delegation of tasks.

_____

_____

_____

3. List and describe two responsibilities of the nursing assistant regarding delegation of tasks.

_____

_____

_____

Activity J *Fill in the blanks using the words given in brackets.*

[written, delegation, accountability, practice]

1. State laws form the basis of the state's standards of _____ for nursing.

2. State laws ensure _____ and responsibility on the part of licensed nurses.

3. Each health care facility has _____ policies about delegation of tasks.

4. _____ of a task may depend on the patient's medical condition.

Activity K *Think About It! Briefly answer the following questions in the space provided.*

A nurse has delegated the task of performing a sterile dressing change to a nursing assistant.

1. What factors should the nursing assistant consider before accepting the assignment?

_____

_____

_____

2. What should the nursing assistant do if training has not been provided for the task delegated?

_____

_____

_____

COMMUNICATION IN THE ADVANCED CARE SETTING

Key Learning Point

- Special considerations regarding communication when working in an advanced care setting

Activity L *Think About It! Briefly answer the following questions in the space provided.*

1. Why are rephrasing and asking open-ended questions of patients important?

   _____

   _____

   _____

2. What steps can a nursing assistant take to ensure accurate and factual reporting of information?

   _____

   _____

   _____

3. A nursing assistant is caring for a patient who is unable to hear or understand him. What steps can the nursing assistant take so that the communication between them is clear?

   _____

   _____

   _____

Activity M *Place an "X" next to the correct method of documenting patient information.*

1. _____ Write neatly with dark ink.

2. _____ Refer to the patient by first name only.

3. _____ Use only facility-approved abbreviations.

4. _____ Ensure that all entries are signed and dated appropriately.

5. _____ Write down vital sign measurements after leaving the patient's room.

SUMMARY

Activity N *Match the terms in Column A with their descriptions in Column B.*

Column A

_____ 1. Advanced care settings

_____ 2. Humanistic health care

_____ 3. The nursing assistant

_____ 4. Government regulations

_____ 5. The nurse

Column B

a. Must receive additional training to perform advanced skills

b. Ensure that health care provided by facilities is safe and of high quality

c. Provide a high level of care and monitoring for patients

d. Responsible for delegating tasks and providing adequate supervision

e. Acting with compassion, kindness, and respect

CHAPTER 2

Sterile Technique

PREVENTING HEALTH CARE–ASSOCIATED INFECTIONS

Key Learning Points

- The proper use of sterile technique is critical
- Definition of *sterile technique* and when it is used

Activity A *Fill in the blanks using the words given in brackets.*

[sterile, disinfection, pathogens, sanitization]

1. Skin that is without cuts, scrapes, or wounds

   physically prevents _____ from entering the body.

2. Handwashing is an example of _____ technique for medical asepsis.

3. General _____ uses chemicals to reduce the number of microbes on a surface to a safe level.

4. When a patient must undergo an invasive procedure or has a medical condition that

   disrupts the skin, _____ technique is used.

Activity B *Think About It! Briefly answer the following question in the space provided.*

People who are being cared for in health care settings are at risk for health care–associated infections (HAIs). List situations that would increase a patient's risk for getting an HAI.

_____

_____

Activity C *Place an "X" next to each correct answer for the following question.*

1. Sterile technique must be used to prevent the patient from getting a health care–associated infection (HAI). Which of the following procedures require the use of sterile technique?

   a. _____ Assisting with meals

   b. _____ Giving injections

   c. _____ Starting intravenous (IV) lines

   d. _____ Inserting urinary catheters

   e. _____ Obtaining blood pressure

Activity D *Identify the procedure being performed in the image.*

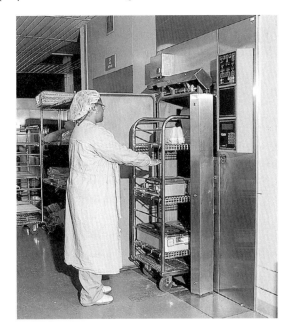

_____

5

STERILE EQUIPMENT AND SUPPLIES

Key Learning Points

- Classification of medical equipment according to disinfection or sterilization requirements
- The processes of high-level disinfection and sterilization and the difference between the two
- Packaging of sterile items and supplies
- How to verify that the contents of a sterile package are sterile
- How to properly handle and store sterile packages to maintain their sterility

Activity E *Match the types of disinfection and sterilization given in Column A with their techniques given in Column B.*

Column A

_____ 1. High-level disinfection can be achieved by
_____ 2. Prepackaged sterile items are sterilized by
_____ 3. Instruments and equipment are sterilized on-site by

Column B

a. Using ionizing radiation
b. Using heat (steam under pressure)
c. Using very strong chemicals

Activity F *Fill in the blanks using the words given in brackets.*

[peel, endospore, boiling]

1. High-level disinfection can also be achieved by _____ an item for 10 to 20 minutes.

2. Small items may be packaged in combination plastic and paper wrappers known as _____ pouches.

3. Some types of bacteria can surround themselves with a protective shell, called a/an _____.

Activity G *The following are examples of medical equipment. Place a "C" next to critical items, an "S" next to semi-critical items, and an "N" next to noncritical items.*

1. _____ Vascular and urinary catheters
2. _____ Endoscopes
3. _____ Food utensils
4. _____ Needles
5. _____ Respiratory therapy equipment
6. _____ Implants

Activity H *Select the single best answer for each of the following questions.*

1. Which of the following items would require general disinfection?
   a. Surgical instruments and supplies
   b. Bedside tables
   c. Anesthesia equipment
   d. Vaginal speculums

2. Which of the following items would require high-level disinfection?
   a. Bed frames
   b. Crutches
   c. Bed linens
   d. Bronchoscopes

Activity I *Match the procedures for high-level disinfection and sterilization of reusable items given in Column A with their correct steps given in Column B.*

Column A

_____ 1. Before sterilizing or disinfecting any item
_____ 2. Items that are to be soaked in a high-level disinfecting liquid
_____ 3. Items that have been soaked in a high-level disinfecting liquid

Column B

a. Allowed to dry and cool before they are handled
b. Require a longer sterilizing cycle in a steam sterilizer
c. Cleaned thoroughly to remove residue (such as blood or tissue)
d. Rinsed thoroughly with sterile water before being used

_____ **4.** Items with hollow passageways or that are made of porous materials

e. Dried thoroughly before placing them in the liquid

_____ **5.** Wrapped items that have been steam-sterilized

Activity J *Select the single best answer for each of the following questions.*

1. Which of the following describes sterile supplies that are packaged by the manufacturer?

  a. They are wrapped in fabric and then in paper.

  b. They are wrapped in paper and then in fabric.

  c. They are wrapped in fabric and then in plastic.

  d. They are wrapped in paper and then in plastic.

2. One advantage of an envelope-wrapped package is that it _____.

  a. Allows the user to peel open the package in one motion.

  b. Allows the user to create a sterile field with the packaging material.

  c. Always uses fabric or linen wrapping material.

  d. Creates a moisture-proof seal to protect contents from contamination.

3. Why is it important to rotate sterile items by placing more recently purchased items behind or under older ones?

  a. To use older supplies before newer ones

  b. To discard old items easily when they expire

  c. To preserve new items for emergencies

  d. To protect new items from contamination

4. Which of the following does the indicator strip on a sterile package suggest?

  a. Guidelines for using the item

  b. Instructions for safe disposal of the item

  c. Evidence of sterilization of the item

  d. Expiration date of the sterile item

Activity K *Think About It! Briefly answer the following question in the space provided.*

A nursing assistant is setting up supplies for a urinary catheterization procedure on a patient. The supplies are in sterile, commercially prepared packages. What should the nursing assistant check for before using the commercially packaged items?

_____

_____

USING STERILE TECHNIQUE

Key Learning Points

- Guidelines that health care workers follow to maintain sterility of equipment, supplies, and the work surface when using sterile technique
- Proper techniques for creating a sterile field using an envelope-wrapped package and using a sterile drape
- Proper techniques for adding envelope-wrapped sterile supplies to a sterile field and for adding sterile supplies that are contained in a peel pouch to a sterile field
- Proper technique for pouring liquid into a sterile container
- Methods used to move sterile supplies around on a sterile field
- Proper technique for putting on and removing sterile gloves

Activity L *Match the steps for using sterile gloves given in Column A with their corresponding actions given in Column B.*

Column A

_____ **1.** Verify that the gloves are sterile.

_____ **2.** Open the inner package.

_____ **3.** Think "glove to glove."

_____ **4.** Think "skin to skin."

Column B

a. Grasp the other glove with one gloved hand to pull it off.

b. Slip two fingers of the ungloved hand under the cuff of the remaining glove.

c. Look for the statement on the outside of the package.

d. Grasp the center flaps and pull them open to the sides.

Activity M *Select the single best answer for each of the following questions.*

1. Which of the following guidelines apply when using sterile technique?

   a. Create the sterile field as close as possible to the time of the procedure.

   b. Avoid using an over-bed table as work surface.

   c. Cover a sterile field for use at a later time if not required immediately.

   d. Keep the front of the uniform at least 5 inches away from the sterile field.

2. Which of the following should be used as a sterile field in case an envelope-wrapped sterile package is not available?

   a. An over-bed table

   b. A paper towel

   c. A clean white towel

   d. A sterile paper drape

3. Which of the following is considered correct technique when creating a sterile field using a sterile drape?

   a. Use water and paper towels to clean the work surface.

   b. Make sure the drape does not touch the arms or uniform.

   c. Shake the sterile drape open if it does not unfold properly.

   d. Grasp the center of the drape and lift it up straight from its package.

4. Which of the following sterile solutions would be manufactured in a single-use bottle?

   a. Hydrogen peroxide

   b. Betadine

   c. Normal saline

   d. Alcohol

5. Which of the following is the correct method of pouring a sterile solution into a sterile container?

   a. Hold the tip of the bottle about 4 to 6 inches above the sterile basin.

   b. Hold the tip of the bottle so it touches the tip of the sterile basin.

   c. Hold the basin by its edge and tilt it slightly while pouring the solution.

   d. Hold the basin 4 to 6 inches above the work surface to pour the solution.

6. Which of the following best describes the term "lipping" when using multiple-use bottles?

   a. Removing the cap of the bottle to pour solution

   b. Pouring a small amount of solution into the waste container

   c. Re-capping the bottle after pouring solution

   d. Discarding old solution from a multiple-use bottle

Activity N *Figures of devices used for handling sterile equipment are given below. Identify the equipment.*

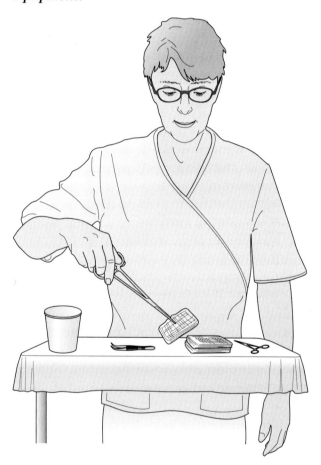

1. _____

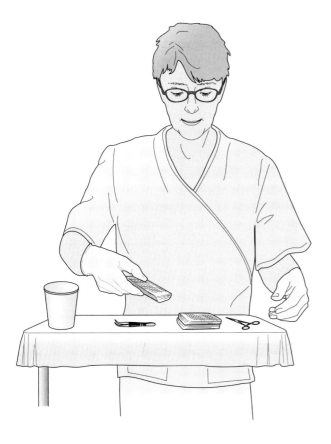

2.

_____

Activity O *The following are examples of events that may occur while setting up or handling sterile supplies. Place an "X" next to events that warrant discarding the item and a "U" next to events that allow the use of the sterile item.*

1. _____ Gloves touch an item that is sterile.

2. _____ A non-sterile item touches a sterile item.

3. _____ A peel pouch tears evenly along the edges.

4. _____ The patient reaches up and touches the sterile supplies.

5. _____ A liquid solution is spilled onto a sterile drape.

6. _____ The uniform touches the sterile drape.

Activity P *Match the actions involved in using sterile technique given in Column A with their rationales given in Column B.*

Column A

_____ **1.** Clean and dry the work surface where a sterile field will be created.

_____ **2.** Keep sterile items above waist level or the work surface.

_____ **3.** Unfold the first flap of an envelope-wrapped sterile package away from the body.

_____ **4.** Avoid reaching across a sterile field with bare hands.

_____ **5.** Keep sterile items in the center of the sterile field.

Column B

a. Keeps sterile items in one's line of sight.

b. Moisture could penetrate the sterile paper or cloth drape and contaminate it.

c. The outer 1 inch of the field is not sterile because of contact with the work surface and ungloved hands.

d. Small flakes of skin or hair can fall onto the sterile field below and contaminate it.

e. This prevents the user from reaching across the sterile field and contaminating it.

Activity Q *Think About It! Briefly answer the following question in the space provided.*

While opening supplies for a sterile dressing change, the nursing assistant accidentally touches the sterile item as she is opening it and then drops it onto the sterile field. What should the nursing assistant do?

_____

_____

_____

Activity R *Match the conditions involved in working in a sterile field given in Column A with their appropriate actions given in Column B.*

Column A

_____ **1.** When using transfer forceps

_____ **2.** If you open an item that is not sterile onto a sterile field

_____ **3.** If you accidentally touch something that is not sterile

_____ **4.** If you had a sterile item in your hand when you contaminated your glove

Column B

a. Stop, immediately back away from the sterile field, and change your gloves.

b. Do not place it back on the sterile field.

c. Avoid touching the tip to anything that is not sterile.

d. Discard the sterile field and create a new one.

Activity S *Think About It! Briefly answer the following question in the space provided.*

The nurse asks the nursing assistant to pour sterile solution from a multiple-use bottle into a basin on the sterile field. Briefly list the steps of the procedure.

_____

_____

_____

SUMMARY

Activity T *Fill in the blanks using the words given in brackets.*

[noncritical, microbes, nosocomial, critical, endospores]

1. To prevent a patient from developing a health care–associated infection (HAI), it is necessary to ensure that the equipment, the work surface, the supplies, and the hands of the health care workers performing the procedure are as free of _____ as possible.

2. _____ items penetrate the skin or are placed into body cavities that are normally free of microbes.

3. Semi-critical items must be free of all microbes except for _____ and are processed using high-level disinfection.

4. _____ items only come in contact with intact skin.

5. Health care–associated infections (HAIs) are also called _____ infections.

CHAPTER 5

Advanced Nutrition Skills

ENTERAL NUTRITION

Key Learning Points

- Why enteral nutrition is the next best option when taking food and fluids through the mouth is not possible
- How a nasogastric or nasointestinal tube is used to provide enteral nutrition
- Risks associated with the use of a nasogastric or nasointestinal tube
- The proper technique for removing a nasogastric tube
- How a gastrostomy or jejunostomy tube is used to provide enteral nutrition
- Three ways of administering enteral nutrition
- The different schedules that are used to administer enteral nutrition
- The different ways enteral feeding formulas may be packaged
- The nursing assistant's role in caring for a person who is receiving enteral nutrition
- Complications that can occur when a person is receiving enteral nutrition and ways the nursing team helps to prevent these complications from occurring
- Signs and symptoms that a person who is receiving enteral nutrition may have that should be reported to the nurse right away

Activity A *Fill in the blanks using the words given in brackets.*

[chyme, hydration, enteral, absorption]

1. Proper nutrition and _____ are essential for health and healing.

2. The transfer of nutrients from the digestive tract into the bloodstream is called _____.

3. _____ is the liquid substance produced by digestion of the food in the stomach.

4. With _____ nutrition, food is placed directly into the stomach or intestines.

Activity B *Select the single best answer for each of the following questions.*

1. Which of the following normal processes does not occur in a person receiving enteral nutrition?
   a. Absorption
   b. Digestion
   c. Excretion
   d. Ingestion

2. Which of the following is not a possible complication of using a nasogastric or nasointestinal tube?
   a. Pressure sores inside the nose
   b. Aspiration of feeding formula
   c. Crusting of mucus around the nostrils
   d. Excessive salivation

Activity C *Think About It! Briefly answer the following question in the space provided.*

A nursing assistant is caring for a patient who is being fed through a nasogastric tube. The nursing assistant needs to confirm that the tube is in the correct position before administering formula through the nasogastric tube. The nursing assistant asks the nurse to confirm that the tube is in the right place. List three methods the nurse can use to check the placement of the tube.

_____

_____

_____

Activity D *Place an "X" next to each correct answer for the following question.*

1. Which of the following should a nursing assistant check for at the insertion site of a person with a gastrostomy tube?

   a. _____ Leaking formula

   b. _____ Redness

   c. _____ A small amount of mucous

   d. _____ Drainage

   e. _____ Pink, healthy skin

Activity E *Write down the correct order of activities that take place while removing a nasogastric tube in the boxes provided below.*

a. Raise the head of the bed to the semi-Fowler's position.

b. Pull the tube out in one continuous motion.

c. Assist the patient with oral care.

d. Remove the tape from the patient's nose.

e. Ask the person to take a deep breath.

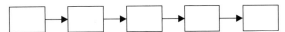

Activity F *Fill in the blanks using the words given in brackets.*

[jejunostomy, nasogastric, percutaneous, gastrostomy]

1. A _____ tube is inserted through the nose, down the throat, and into the stomach.

2. A _____ tube is inserted into the stomach through a surgically made opening in the abdomen.

3. A _____ tube is inserted into a part of the small intestine through a surgically made opening in the abdomen.

4. A _____ endoscopic gastrostomy tube is a special type of gastrostomy tube.

Activity G *Various methods of administering enteral nutrition are shown below. Identify the methods.*

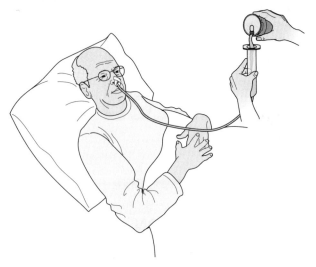

1. _____

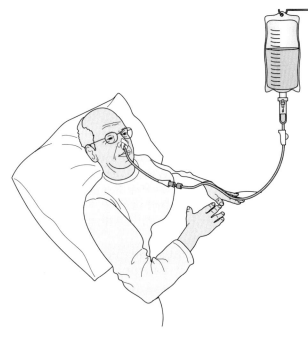

2. _____

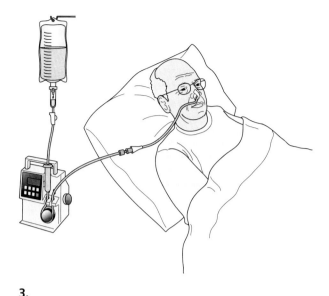

3. _____

Activity H *Match the type of feeding in Column A with its description in Column B.*

Column A

_____ **1.** Bolus intermittent feeding

_____ **2.** Intermittent feeding

_____ **3.** Continuous feeding

_____ **4.** Cyclic feeding

Column B

a. The person receives a small amount of formula constanly for 20 to 24 hours a day

b. The person receives a small amount of formula for 8 to 12 hours and then is disconnected from the feeding pump

c. Person receives large amount of formula over a short period of time several times throughout the day and night

d. Person receives a large amount of formula over a large period of time several times throughout the day and night

Activity I *Select the single best answer for the following question.*

1. Which type of feeding provides the maximum amount of calories and nutrition with a minimal amount of complications?
   a. Bolus intermittent feeding
   b. Continuous feeding
   c. Intermittent feeding
   d. Cyclic feeding

Activity J *Think About It! Briefly answer the following question in the space provided.*

Why is it important to check the label on the can, packet, or bottle of formula?

_____

_____

_____

Activity K *Place an "X" next to each correct answer for the following questions.*

1. Which of the following are possible complications for a patient receiving enteral nutrition?
   a. _____ Aspiration
   b. _____ Dehydration
   c. _____ Health care–associated infection
   d. _____ Adequate urine output
   e. _____ Moist mucous membranes

2. Which of the following can be caused by dehydration, if not treated?
   a. _____ Indigestion
   b. _____ Heart dysrhythmia
   c. _____ Kidney failure
   d. _____ Death
   e. _____ Vomiting

Activity L *The following are certain signs that may be observed in a patient. Place an "X" next to signs shown by a patient receiving enteral nutrition that need to be reported to the nurse immediately.*

1. _____ Wheezing
2. _____ Back pain
3. _____ Abdominal pain
4. _____ Dry mucous membranes
5. _____ Vomiting
6. _____ Increased urine output

TOTAL PARENTERAL NUTRITION

Key Learning Points

- How total parenteral nutrition (TPN) differs from enteral nutrition
- Why a person might require TPN
- The nursing assistant's role in caring for a person who is receiving TPN

Activity M *Fill in the blanks using the words given in brackets.*

[central, hypoglycemia, sterile, hyperalimentation]

1. Total parenteral nutrition is also called

   _____.

2. The total parenteral nutrition (TPN) solution is made by a pharmacist under _____ conditions.

3. A nursing assistant must make sure to check the dressing over the _____ line insertion site when caring for a patient who is receiving TPN.

4. A patient can develop _____ after being taken off TPN.

Activity N *Select the single best answer for the following question.*

1. When should people receiving total parenteral nutrition (TPN) have their blood glucose levels checked?
   a. On completion of TPN
   b. Every 6 hours
   c. Every 12 hours
   d. Every 36 hours

Activity O *Place an "X" next to each correct answer for the following question.*

1. A large vein located at which of the following locations is used to insert a catheter for total parenteral nutrition (TPN)?
   a. _____ Shoulder
   b. _____ Chest
   c. _____ Hips
   d. _____ Neck
   e. _____ Groin

Activity P *Think About It! Briefly answer the following question in the space provided.*

A nursing assistant is caring for a patient with head injuries after a motor vehicle accident. The doctor has ordered total parenteral nutrition (TPN) for the patient. What are the reasons TPN might be necessary?

_____

_____

_____

MONITORING BLOOD GLUCOSE LEVELS

Key Learning Points

- Why a person might need to have his or her blood glucose levels monitored
- The proper technique for monitoring a person's blood glucose level

Activity Q *Fill in the blanks using the words given in brackets.*

[glucagon, glucose, hypoglycemia, insulin, hyperglycemia]

1. _____ is the body's most basic source of fuel.

2. The pancreas produces the hormone _____, which releases glycogen into the bloodstream.

3. _____ and glucagon work together to keep the body's blood glucose levels stable.

4. _____ occurs when the blood glucose level is excessively high.

5. _____ occurs when the blood glucose level is excessively low.

Activity R *Place an "X" next to each correct answer for the following questions.*

1. What are the long-term complications of untreated hyperglycemia?
   a. _____ Nerve damage
   b. _____ Blindness
   c. _____ Deafness
   d. _____ Arterial ulcers
   e. _____ Kidney disease

2. Which of the following things should a nursing assistant keep in mind when performing a quality control (QC) test on a blood glucose meter?
   a. _____ Check that the solution is not past the expiration date.
   b. _____ Check that the solution has the minimum glucose content.
   c. _____ Shake the solution thoroughly.
   d. _____ Record the results of the QC test.
   e. _____ Check how many patients need their blood glucose levels monitored.

Activity S *Select the single best answer for the following question.*

1. Which of the following blood glucose levels needs to be reported to the nurse immediately?

   a. 65 mg/dL

   b. 75 mg/dL

   c. 95 mg/dL

   d. 115 mg/dL

Activity T *Write down the correct order of activities that take place while monitoring blood glucose levels in the boxes provided below.*

a. Gently touch the person's finger to the testing strip.

b. Insert the testing strip into the meter.

c. Apply pressure to the puncture site using a tissue or cotton ball.

d. Press the lancet straight down to pierce the person's skin.

e. Help the person to wash his or her hands with soap and water.

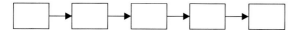

Activity U *Think About It! Briefly answer the following question in the space provided.*

Why is it important to use a new lancet for each patient?

_____

_____

_____

SUMMARY

Activity V *Fill in the blanks using the words given in brackets.*

[pathogens, bacteria, humidity]

1. Wearing gloves when obtaining a blood glucose sample helps limit the exposure to bloodborne _____.

2. The testing strips are sensitive to light and _____.

3. _____ can increase rapidly in enteral feeding formulas.

Advanced Vascular Access Skills

VENIPUNCTURE

Key Learning Points

- Using a needle and syringe or a vacuum tube system to obtain a blood specimen
- Safety precautions that must be followed when using a tourniquet
- Veins commonly used for venipuncture
- Characteristics of a suitable vein for venipuncture
- Proper technique for performing venipuncture using a vacuum tube system

Activity A *Fill in the blanks using the words given in brackets.*

[phlebotomist, blood, phlebotomy, venipuncture, vascular]

1. _____ is the life-giving fluid of our bodies.

2. The _____ system, which is made up of the blood vessels, transports the blood throughout the body.

3. _____ is the act of obtaining blood from a vein for therapeutic or diagnostic purpose.

4. The use of a needle to pierce a vein and withdraw blood is called _____.

5. A _____ is a specialist who is responsible for collecting blood specimens.

Activity B *Place an "X" next to each correct answer for the following question.*

1. A syringe is a device used to inject or withdraw fluids. Which of the following are the parts of a syringe?
   a. _____ Plunger
   b. _____ Barrel
   c. _____ Tip
   d. _____ Needle
   e. _____ Hub

Activity C *Fill in the blanks using the words given in brackets.*

[shaft, needle, vacuum, bevel]

1. A slender, hollow steel tube with a sharp end used for piercing is called a _____.

2. The slanted end of the needle is called the _____.

3. The _____ of the syringe can be long or short and varies in diameter.

4. Pulling back on the plunger creates a _____ in the syringe.

Activity D *Identify the object shown in the figure.*

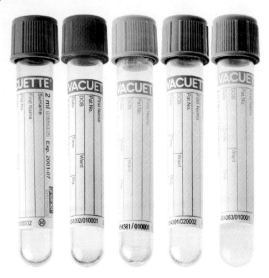

_____

Activity E *Match each component of a vacuum tube system given in Column A with its use or description given in Column B.*

Column A

_____ **1.** Long bevel

_____ **2.** Additives

_____ **3.** Vacuum tube

_____ **4.** Short bevel

_____ **5.** Multisample needle

Column B

a. A special needle with bevels on both ends

b. Used to pierce the stopper on the vacuum tube

c. A sealed glass or plastic tube from which air has been removed

d. Used to prevent the blood sample from clotting

e. Used to enter the vein

Activity F *Select the single best answer for the following question.*

1. What advantage does a vacuum tube system have over a needle and syringe for drawing a blood specimen?

  a. It keeps the blood from spilling out of the tube.

  b. It keeps the blood collected for testing sterile.

  c. It allows for multiple specimens without removing the needle from the person's arm.

  d. It uses a smaller needle and is therefore less painful for the patient.

Activity G *Fill in the blanks using the words given in brackets.*

[venous, arterial, radial, venipuncture]

1. A long, flat strip of stretchy latex or vinyl used during _____ is called a tourniquet.

2. A tourniquet blocks _____ blood flow, causing the veins to bulge.

3. A tight tourniquet may block _____ blood flow, causing tissue or nerve damage.

4. The _____ pulse cannot be felt if the tourniquet is too tight.

Activity H *The veins that are commonly used for venipuncture are shown in the figure below. Identify the veins.*

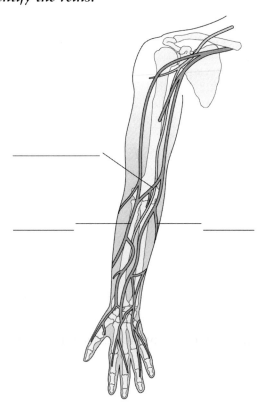

Activity I *Select the single best answer for each of the following questions.*

1. Which one of the following complications can occur if blood is drawn from an artery?
   a. Clot formation
   b. Air embolism
   c. Pulmonary embolism
   d. Meningitis

2. Which of the following is the best vein to use for venipuncture?
   a. A vein that pulsates
   b. A vein that feels firm and full, like a cooked spaghetti noodle
   c. A vein that is flat when the tourniquet is on
   d. A vein that is hard and cord-like

Activity J *Place an "X" next to each correct answer for the following question.*

1. The veins in the inner aspect of the elbow are most frequently used for venipuncture. Which of the following conditions can make the vein hard to find?
   a. _____ Obesity
   b. _____ Chemotherapy
   c. _____ Dehydration
   d. _____ Chest pain
   e. _____ Difficulty breathing

Activity K *Think About It! Briefly answer the following questions in the space provided.*

1. What is a hematoma?

   _____

   _____

   _____

2. What should the nursing assistant do if a hematoma starts to form while drawing blood?

   _____

   _____

   _____

3. What precautions should be taken to reduce the risk of infection during venipuncture?

   _____

   _____

   _____

Activity L *Write down the correct order of venipuncture in the boxes provided below.*

1. Insert the needle into the vein at a 15- to 30-degree angle to the skin.
2. Hold the needle with the bevel pointing up.
3. Fully extend the patient's arm and keep it pointed slightly downward.
4. Support the patient's arm on a firm surface, such as the over-bed table.
5. Place the patient in a supine position.

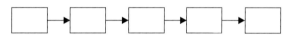

INTRAVENOUS THERAPY

Key Learning Points

- Uses of intravenous therapy
- Difference between a peripheral line and a central line
- Role of the nursing assistant in caring for a person who is receiving intravenous therapy
- Proper technique for removing a peripheral line

Activity M *Fill in the blanks using the words given in brackets.*

[infiltration, phlebitis, thrombophlebitis]

1. Inflammation of the vein is called

   _____.

2. Formation of blood clots within the vein is termed _____.

3. The leaking of intravenous fluid into the tissues around the vein is called _____.

Activity N *Place an "X" next to each correct answer for the following question.*

1. Which of the following complications may occur because of peripheral line insertion?

   a. _____ Pulmonary embolism

   b. _____ Pulmonary hypertension

   c. _____ Thrombophlebitis

   d. _____ Emphysema

   e. _____ Stroke

Activity O *Think About It! Briefly answer the following question in the space provided.*

List observations that the nursing assistant should immediately report when caring for a patient with a peripheral line.

_____

_____

_____

Activity P *A central line is a large intravenous catheter that is inserted into a large vein in the neck, chest, or groin and ends in one of the two large veins that empties directly into the heart. Identify the type of central line shown below.*

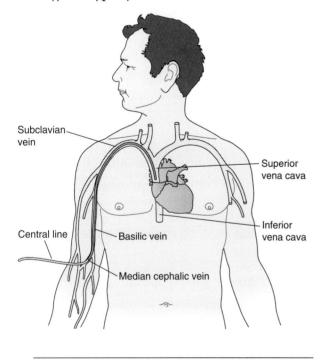

Subclavian vein

Central line

Basilic vein

Median cephalic vein

Superior vena cava

Inferior vena cava

_____

_____

_____

Activity Q *Select the single best answer for the following question.*

1. Which of the following is an advantage of administering total parenteral nutrition through a central line?

   a. Prevents rapid dilution of the solution by the blood

   b. Prevents the lining of the veins from becoming irritated

   c. Prevents the ventricles from filling all the way with blood

   d. Affects the amount of blood that is sent out to the body

Activity R *Fill in the blanks using the words given in brackets.*

[bacteremia, fungemia, endocarditis]

1. Presence of bacteria in the bloodstream is called _____.

2. Infection of the endocardium is called _____.

3. Presence of fungi in the bloodstream is called _____.

Activity S *Place an "X" next to each correct answer for the following question.*

1. Which of the following complications can occur in a patient with a central line?

   a. _____ Vomiting

   b. _____ Bloodstream infection

   c. _____ Bronchitis

   d. _____ Air embolism

   e. _____ Endocarditis

Activity T *Think About It! Briefly answer the following questions in the space provided.*

1. When caring for a patient who has a central intravenous line, the nursing assistant should take care to not

_____

_____

_____

2. What observations should the nursing assistant immediately report to the nurse when caring for a patient with a central line?

_____

_____

_____

SUMMARY

Activity U *Fill in the blanks using the words given in brackets.*

[vacuum, venipuncture, peripheral]

1. Veins, not arteries, are used for _____.

2. A _____ tube system is most often used to collect blood specimens.

3. A _____ line has a short catheter with a small diameter.

Activity V *Think About It! Briefly answer the following question in the space provided.*

What is intravenous therapy, and how can it be delivered?

_____

_____

_____

Activity W *Select the single best answer for the following question.*

1. Which of the following is an appropriate site for peripheral line insertion?
    a. Neck
    b. Chest
    c. Groin
    d. Hand

Activity X *Think About It! Briefly answer the following question in the space provided.*

What are the differences between a peripheral and a central line?

_____

_____

_____

Activity Y *Place an "X" next to each correct answer for the following question.*

1. A central line is a large intravenous catheter that is inserted into a large vein. Which of the following insertion sites may be used for a central line?
    a. _____ Hips
    b. _____ Chest
    c. _____ Groin
    d. _____ Hand
    e. _____ Neck

CHAPTER 9

Care of the Rehabilitation Patient

REHABILITATION: AN OVERVIEW

Key Learning Points

- Major goals of rehabilitation and settings where rehabilitation can take place
- The three phases of the rehabilitation process
- Areas addressed as part of a rehabilitation program
- Responsibilities of key members of the rehabilitation team
- Factors that can affect the outcome of the rehabilitation effort

Activity A *Fill in the blanks using the words given in brackets.*

[disability, chronic, rehabilitation]

1. Restoring and maintaining physical, emotional, and social function is a major

   goal of _____.

2. A condition that results in a loss of function

   is a _____.

3. A _____ condition that progressively worsens may result in a disability.

Activity B *Think About It! Briefly answer the following question in the space provided.*

1. List some conditions that may require rehabilitation in a specialized rehabilitation center.

   _____

   _____

   _____

Activity C *Place an "X" next to each correct answer for the following question.*

1. Which of the following might the patient need in the subacute phase of rehabilitation?

   a. _____ Ventilator support

   b. _____ Vocational counseling

   c. _____ Intravenous fluids

   d. _____ Education about the disability or disorder

   e. _____ Enteral feedings

Activity D *The following are descriptions of phases of rehabilitation. Place an "A" next to descriptions indicating acute phase, an "S" next to descriptions indicating subacute phase, and a "C" next to descriptions indicating chronic phase.*

1. _____ Restores the person's mental health

2. _____ Focuses on stabilizing the person's medical condition

3. _____ Restores the person's ability to communicate

4. _____ Focuses on keeping the person alive

5. _____ Prevents complications associated with immobility

6. _____ Focuses on maintaining the person's ability to move independently

Activity E *Match the health care workers who specialize in rehabilitation given in Column A with their function given in Column B.*

Column A	Column B
_____ **1.** Rehabilitation nurse	**a.** Helps the patient regain or maintain the ability to perform activities of daily living
_____ **2.** Occupational therapist	
_____ **3.** Physical therapist	**b.** Helps the patient regain or maintain strength, endurance, coordination, posture, and flexibility
_____ **4.** Speech therapist	
_____ **5.** Orthotist	**c.** Fits the patient with supportive devices to correct deformity, aid movement, and relieve discomfort
	d. Develops a nursing care plan to maximize the patient's functioning and quality of life
	e. Helps the patient regain or maintain the ability to communicate with others and swallow

Activity F *Think About It! Briefly answer the following question in the space provided.*

1. Give some examples of how a person's attitude and coping skills can affect the rehabilitation effort.

_____

_____

_____

Activity G *Place an "X" next to each correct answer for the following question.*

1. When family members treat a disabled person as a responsible, capable person, they have a positive effect on the person's rehabilitation by helping to:

a. _____ Build self-esteem

b. _____ Promote independence

c. _____ Perform all activities for the patient

d. _____ Promote dependence on others

e. _____ Assist in rehabilitation

Activity H *Think About It! Briefly answer the following question in the space provided.*

1. What factors can affect the outcome of a rehabilitation effort?

_____

_____

_____

REHABILITATION: SPECIFIC SITUATIONS

Key Learning Points

- The nursing assistant's role in caring for a person with a spinal cord injury during the acute, subacute, and chronic phases of rehabilitation
- The nursing assistant's role in caring for a person with a traumatic brain injury (TBI) during the acute, subacute, and chronic phases of rehabilitation
- The nursing assistant's role in caring for a person who has had a stroke during the acute, subacute, and chronic phases of rehabilitation
- The nursing assistant's role in caring for a person with a cardiovascular disorder during the acute, subacute, and chronic phases of rehabilitation
- The nursing assistant's role in caring for a person with a musculoskeletal disorder during the acute, subacute, and chronic phases of rehabilitation
- The nursing assistant's role in caring for a person with a burn injury during the acute, subacute, and chronic phases of rehabilitation
- Why an elderly person might require rehabilitation

Activity I *Fill in the blanks using the words given in brackets.*

[tetraplegia, paraplegia, severity, brain]

1. The spinal cord is the line of communication between the _____ and the rest of the body.

2. The disability that results from a spinal cord injury depends on the _____ of the injury.

3. A person who has a spinal cord injury at level T1 and above will most likely have _____.

4. People with injuries below the level of T1 will most likely have _____.

Activity J *Identify the device in the figure and explain its use.*

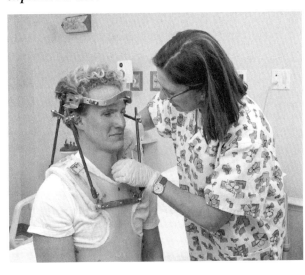

_____

_____

_____

Activity K *Think About It! Briefly answer the following question in the space provided.*

What does the chronic phase of rehabilitation of the patient with a spinal cord injury focus on?

_____

_____

_____

Activity L *Match the forms of traumatic brain injury given in Column A with their descriptions given in Column B.*

Column A	Column B
___ 1. Temporary change in mental status caused by head trauma	a. Subdural hematoma
___ 2. Bruise on the brain that occurs when the brain tissue hits the skull	b. Epidural hematoma
___ 3. Blood collects between the skull and the dura mater	c. Cerebral contusion
___ 4. Blood collects between the dura mater and the arachnoid mater	d. Concussion

Activity M *Fill in the blanks using the words given in brackets.*

[dysphagia, brain, recovery, hemiplegia, skull]

1. The intracranial pressure (ICP) is the pressure in the space between the _____ and the brain.

2. An increase in the ICP can crush the _____ tissue.

3. Difficulty in swallowing is known as _____.

4. Paralysis on one side of the body is known as _____.

5. The Rancho Los Amigos Scale is used by the rehabilitation team to identify the stages of _____ in a patient with a traumatic brain injury.

Activity N *Think About It! Briefly answer the following questions in the space provided.*

1. List the three different categories evaluated by the Glasgow Coma Scale (GCS).

_____

_____

_____

2. How can the level of impairment for a patient be evaluated from his or her total score on the GCS?

_____

_____

_____

3. List four observations that the nursing assistant should immediately report to the nurse when caring for a patient with a head injury.

_____

_____

_____

4. What is the focus of rehabilitation during the chronic phase in the patient with a head injury?

_____

_____

_____

Activity O *Fill in the blanks using the words given in brackets.*

[hemorrhagic, cerebrovascular, ischemic]

1. A/An _____ accident occurs when part of the brain is deprived of blood flow, causing the tissue to die.

2. A/An _____ stroke occurs when an artery in the brain is partially or completely blocked.

3. A/An _____ stroke occurs when an artery in the brain bursts.

Activity P *Place an "X" next to each correct answer for the following questions.*

1. Which of the following are common disabilities that may result from a stroke?

   a. _____ Hemiplegia

   b. _____ Aphasia

   c. _____ Dysphagia

   d. _____ Vomiting

   e. _____ Paraplegia

2. Which of the following are signs of aspiration that the nursing assistant should report to the nurse immediately?

   a. _____ Noisy breathing

   b. _____ Cyanosis of the lips

   c. _____ Easy bruising

   d. _____ Tar-like black stool

   e. _____ Coughing

Activity Q *Think About It! Briefly answer the following question in the space provided.*

List four observations that the nursing assistant should report immediately to the nurse when caring for a patient who has had a stroke.

_____

_____

_____

Activity R *Write down the correct sequence of the events that occur during myocardial infarction in the boxes provided below.*

1. The heart pumps less effectively.

2. Blood is prevented from reaching certain parts of the heart.

3. The heart muscles die due to lack of oxygen.

4. The coronary arteries become completely blocked.

□ → □ → □ → □

Activity S *Fill in the blanks using the words given in brackets.*

[angiogram, stent, angiography]

1. A/An _____ is used to determine if one or more coronary arteries are blocked.

2. A special dye injected through the catheter makes the vessels visible on the x-ray, which is called a/an _____.

3. Balloon angioplasty may be done along with placement of a small coiled wire called _____.

Activity T *Think About It! Briefly answer the following question in the space provided.*

A nursing assistant is caring for a patient who has had cardiac catheterization. The patient is instructed to remain still and quiet in the bed for several hours. List ways in which the nursing assistant may need to assist the patient.

_____

_____

_____

Activity U *Place an "X" next to each correct answer for the following questions.*

1. Which of the following are the signs of good blood flow to the leg below the puncture site after cardiac catheterization?
   a. _____ Pulse felt on top of the foot
   b. _____ Cold, bluish, or gray legs
   c. _____ Pulse felt on the inside of the ankle
   d. _____ Warm legs
   e. _____ Complaints of numbness

2. Which of the following may be used to restore the heart's normal rhythm if the patient goes into cardiac arrest during a myocardial infarction?
   a. _____ Cardiopulmonary resuscitation
   b. _____ Emergency medications
   c. _____ Defibrillation
   d. _____ ECG monitor
   e. _____ Pulse oximeter

Activity V *Think About It! Briefly answer the following question in the space provided.*

List three observations the nursing assistant should report immediately to the nurse when caring for a patient who is recovering from myocardial infarction.

_____

_____

_____

Activity W *Identify the type of fracture shown in the figure below.*

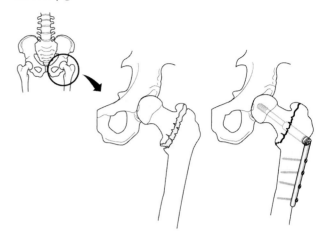

_____

Activity X *Select the single best answer for each of the following questions.*

1. Which of the following factors increases a person's risk of a hip fracture?
   a. Osteoporosis
   b. Arthritis
   c. Diabetes
   d. Deep venous thrombosis

2. Which of the following is a complication of immobility in a patient with a hip fracture?
   a. Osteoporosis
   b. Pneumonia
   c. Bone cancer
   d. Tissue swelling

3. Which of the following complications can occur from a hip fracture and cause a person to go into shock?
   a. Bleeding
   b. Clot formation
   c. Poor circulation
   d. Swelling

4. Which of the following is used to reduce and stabilize most hip fractures?
   a. Splints
   b. Plaster casts
   c. Plates, screws, and pins
   d. Traction

Activity Y *Fill in the blanks using the words given in brackets.*

[blood, circulation, tissue]

1. _____ is collected in the tissues around the fracture.

2. _____ swelling can compress nerves or blood vessels, or both.

3. The person's lower legs and feet are monitored for signs of poor _____.

Activity Z *Select the single best answer for the following question.*

1. Which of the following serious complications can result from clot formation in the lower leg?
   a. Myocardial infraction
   b. Pulmonary embolism
   c. Hemorrhage
   d. Coronary artery disease

Activity AA *Place an "X" next to each correct answer for the following question.*

1. Which of the following are signs of deep venous thrombosis that the nursing assistant should report to the nurse?
   a. _____ Warmth
   b. _____ Redness
   c. _____ Numbness
   d. _____ Swelling
   e. _____ Tingling sensation

Activity AB *Think About It! Briefly answer the following question in the space provided.*

What are the goals of chronic rehabilitation in a patient with a hip fracture?

_____

_____

_____

Activity AC *Fill in the blanks using the words given in brackets.*

[trauma, amputation, diabetes]

1. _____ is the removal of a body part, usually all or part of an arm or leg.

2. Foot problems related to _____ are very common and account for many amputations.

3. Amputation may be necessary as a result of _____.

Activity AD *Place an "X" next to each correct answer for the following question.*

1. Which of the following are signs of infection that the nursing assistant should report to the nurse when caring for a patient with amputation?
   a. _____ Foul-smelling wound discharge
   b. _____ Purulent wound drainage
   c. _____ Increased pain at the wound site
   d. _____ Increased bleeding
   e. _____ Calf tenderness in one leg

Activity AE *Fill in the blanks using the words given in brackets.*

[wrapping, positioning, compression]

1. _____ is used to keep the muscles and tendons from shortening.

2. _____ the end of the stump with elastic bandages helps to shape the stump.

3. The stump is wrapped with _____ bandages.

Activity AF *Select the single best answer for the following question.*

1. Which of the following is a type of second-degree burn?
   a. Superficial burn
   b. Full-thickness burn
   c. Deep partial-thickness burn
   d. Superficial partial-thickness burn

Activity AG *Fill in the blanks using the words given in brackets.*

[kidneys, microbes, contractures, fluid]

1. _____ may be lost through the burnt tissue.

2. The _____ may not function due to the shock associated with the injury.

3. Visitors may have to wear protective clothing to limit the patient's exposure to _____.

4. The patient performs range-of-motion exercises during the subacute phase of rehabilitation to help prevent _____.

Activity AH *Think About It! Briefly answer the following question in the space provided.*

What type of procedures may be necessary for a patient with severe burns to help remove dead tissue?

_____

_____

_____

Activity AI *Select the single best answer for the following question.*

1. Which of the following may develop as a result of damage to the tendons and muscles?
   a. Contractures
   b. Amputation
   c. Osteoarthritis
   d. Osteoporosis

Activity AJ *Fill in the blanks using the words given in brackets.*

[hospital, function, rehabilitation]

1. Geriatric rehabilitation programs focus on helping the person regain or maintain _____ and independence.

2. The _____ effort focuses on helping the person to regain strength.

3. Rehabilitation begins in the _____ as soon as the person's medical condition is stabilized.

SUMMARY

Activity AK *Select the single best answer for the following question.*

1. Which of the following conditions can result in a partial or total loss of function or sensation, or both, below the level of the injury?
   a. Traumatic brain injuries
   b. Cardiovascular disorders
   c. Spinal cord injuries
   d. Musculoskeletal disorders

CHAPTER 10

Care of the Surgical Patient

WHAT WILL YOU LEARN?

Key Learning Points

- Reasons surgery may be needed and settings where surgery may take place
- Three phases of surgical care

Activity A *Fill in the blanks using the words given in brackets.*

[hospital, elective, reconstructive]

1. Surgery can be _____ if the person's health is not immediately threatened if the surgery is not performed right away.

2. In the past, most surgeries were performed in the _____ .

3. Many surgeons, especially those specializing in plastic and _____ surgery, may perform procedures in an operating room located in their office or clinic.

Activity B *Select the single best answer for each of the following questions.*

1. A surgical procedure for a condition in which the person's health will suffer if the procedure is not performed within a few days or weeks is considered:
   a. Elective
   b. Definitive
   c. Urgent
   d. Emergent

2. Which of the following is an example of palliative surgery?
   a. Surgery to reduce a cancerous mass
   b. Cardiac bypass surgery
   c. Cleft lip repair
   d. Diagnostic laparoscopy

Activity C *Match the type of surgery given in Column A with its purpose or reason it is done given in Column B.*

Column A	Column B
____ 1. Diagnostic	a. To look inside the body of a person with a significant problem when the doctors do not know exactly what is causing the problem
____ 2. Exploratory	
____ 3. Palliative	b. To relieve uncomfortable symptoms of disease; the surgery is not a cure
____ 4. Cosmetic	
____ 5. Definitive	c. To remove or replace tissue to restore function
	d. To change a person's appearance
	e. To remove tissue from the person's body to determine whether a person has a certain medical condition

Activity D *Think About It! Briefly answer the following question in the space provided.*

List the three phases of care for a person having surgery.

_____

_____

_____

PRE-OPERATIVE PHASE

Key Learning Point

■ Preparations necessary to physically prepare a patient for surgery and the nursing assistant's role in these preparations

Activity E *Fill in the blanks using the words given in brackets.*

[clippers, urinary, physically]

1. In the pre-operative phase, the doctor usually orders tests to assess the functioning of the person's cardiovascular, respiratory, and

   _____ systems.

2. On the day of the surgery, many actions are

   taken to _____ prepare the patient for the procedure.

3. Body hair should be removed using

   disposable _____ instead of a razor.

Activity F *Think About It! Briefly answer the following question in the space provided.*

List four common pre-operative tasks that a nursing assistant may be responsible for assisting the patient with on the day of surgery.

_____

_____

_____

Activity G *Select the single best answer for the following question.*

1. A surgical procedure is scheduled for a person who takes daily medications in the morning. Because the person is to be NPO, how might the doctor request that the patient take the medication?

   a. 3 or 4 hours before the scheduled time

   b. At midnight the night before surgery

   c. At the normal time with a small sip of water

   d. Early in the morning on the day of surgery

Activity H *Think About It! Briefly answer the following questions in the space provided.*

1. A nursing assistant is helping to prepare a patient for surgery. List two duties of the nursing assistant under each of the following aspects of the pre-operative phase.

   a. Maintaining NPO status

   _____

   _____

   b. Preparing the surgical site

   _____

   _____

   c. Dressing and grooming

   _____

   _____

   d. Assisting with elimination

   _____

   _____

INTRA-OPERATIVE PHASE

Key Learning Points

■ Members of the surgical team
■ Physical environment of the surgical suite
■ Methods that are used to help prevent infection in the surgical suite
■ Hazards that may affect a person working in the surgical suite and measures the nursing assistant can take to avoid these hazards
■ Actions the health care team takes to keep the patient safe during surgery

Activity I *Match the members of the surgical team given in Column A with their responsibilities given in Column B.*

Column A	Column B
_____ **1.** Surgeon	**a.** Administers anesthesia
_____ **2.** Nursing assistant	**b.** Manages the nursing care provided in the operating room
_____ **3.** Scrub person	**c.** Performs surgical procedure
_____ **4.** Circulating nurse	**d.** Assists non-sterile team members with transporting, transferring, and positioning the patient
_____ **5.** Anesthesiologist	**e.** Sets up sterile supplies and instruments

Activity J *Place an "X" next to each correct answer for the following question.*

1. Choose the areas that are usually located in the surgical suite.

   a. _____ Employee dressing rooms

   b. _____ Laboratory

   c. _____ Operating rooms

   d. _____ Sterile supply storage rooms

   e. _____ Visitor cafeteria

Activity K *The surgical suite is divided into three defined zones. The purpose of these zones is to limit the introduction of microbes into the environment. List the three zones of the surgical suite.*

_____

_____

_____

Activity L *Select the single best answer for the following question.*

1. In which area of the surgical suite should the health care members wear masks in addition to surgical scrubs and head coverings?

   a. Semi-restricted zone

   b. Post-anesthesia care unit

   c. Restricted zone

   d. Non-restricted zone

Activity M *The following are the different areas of a surgical suite. Place an "N" next to areas that are non-restricted zone, an "S" next to areas that are semi-restricted, and an "R" next to areas that are restricted.*

1. _____ Pre-operative preparation area

2. _____ Storage rooms for non-sterile supplies

3. _____ Storage room for sterile supplies

4. _____ Post-anesthesia care unit

5. _____ Operating rooms

6. _____ Admissions area

7. _____ Inner hallways

8. _____ Employee dressing rooms

Activity N *Fill in the blanks using the words given in brackets.*

[hood, sterile, infectious]

1. The proper use of scrub attire helps protect the members of the surgical team from exposure to _____ disease.

2. Men with beards or long sideburns should cover them with a surgical _____.

3. The area closely surrounding the operating table and the instrument tables is known as a/an _____ field.

Activity O *Place an "X" next to each correct answer for the following questions.*

1. Which of the following are parts of the scrub attire?
   a. _____ Scrub top and pants
   b. _____ Face shields
   c. _____ Shoe covers
   d. _____ False nails
   e. _____ Exposed jewelry

2. Which of the following health care members are sterile team members?
   a. _____ Scrub person
   b. _____ Anesthesia provider
   c. _____ Circulating nurse
   d. _____ Surgical assistant
   e. _____ Surgeon

Activity P *Think About It! Briefly answer the following question in the space provided.*

List three situations that put a person at a higher-than-average risk for developing an infection after surgery.

_____

_____

_____

Activity Q *Match the following workplace hazards given in Column A with the source of the hazard in Column B.*

Column A

_____ 1. Physical injury
_____ 2. Airborne pathogens
_____ 3. Chemical exposure
_____ 4. Fire
_____ 5. Exposure to radiation

Column B

a. Smoke from electrocautery
b. X-ray equipment
c. Disinfecting and sterilizing agents
d. Wet floors in the operating room
e. Fiber-optic light sources

Activity R *Select the single best answer for each of the following questions.*

1. Which type of anesthesia causes a loss of consciousness?
   a. Regional anesthesia
   b. Topical anesthesia
   c. Local anesthesia
   d. General anesthesia

2. Injecting a numbing medication either into a person's spinal column or a nerve pathway is an example of a _____ anesthetic.
   a. Regional
   b. General
   c. Local
   d. Topical

Activity S *Think About It! Briefly answer the following question in the space provided.*

List four additional tasks that are usually performed to prepare the patient for the surgical procedure after the patient receives the appropriate anesthetic.

_____

_____

_____

Activity T *Select the single best answer for each of the following questions.*

1. Which of the following activities might a nursing assistant be responsible for during the intra-operative phase?
   a. Setting up sterile supplies and instruments for the surgery
   b. Assisting the nurse in completing necessary documentation
   c. Assisting with transferring and positioning the patient
   d. Monitoring the patient's response to anesthesia

2. Before surgery actually begins, a "surgical time-out" is taken. What is the purpose of the surgical time-out?

a. To count sponges and instruments

b. To prevent hypothermia

c. To verify the procedure and surgical site

d. To document pre-operative medications

3. Which of the following methods can be used to help prevent hypothermia in patients during surgical procedures?

a. Using warm irrigation solutions

b. Counting all sponges and sharps

c. Lowering the humidity level

d. Lowering the room temperature

4. Which of the following health care providers is responsible for constantly monitoring the amount of blood the patient loses?

a. Anesthesia care provider

b. Circulating nurse

c. Nursing assistant

d. Surgical assistant

POST-OPERATIVE PHASE

Key Learning Point

■ Three phases of recovery that a patient goes through after surgery and the nursing assistant's role in providing care during these three phases

Activity U *Fill in the blanks using the words given in brackets.*

[hypothermia, oxygen, narcotic, suction]

1. Patients who are recovering from general anesthesia receive supplemental _____ and are connected to a pulse oximeter and an electrocardiography monitor.

2. Warm blankets or forced-air warming units are used to keep the person warm and reverse the effects of _____.

3. _____ medications used during surgery and for pain control can cause the person's respirations to be slow and shallow, limiting his intake of oxygen.

4. _____ equipment should be available for every patient who has just come from the operating room to prevent aspiration in case they vomit.

Activity V *Select the single best answer for each of the following questions.*

1. Which of the following complications might occur in the post-operative phase that could lead to the condition of hypovolemic shock?

a. Hemorrhage

b. A distended bladder

c. Shallow respirations

d. Vomiting

2. Which of the following needs is a priority for a person during phase I of the post-operative phase?

a. Ambulation

b. Nutrition

c. Hygiene

d. Respiration

3. Which one of the following signs may indicate an internal hemorrhage after surgery?

a. Aldrete score of 7 or higher

b. Increased swelling around the surgical site

c. Nausea and vomiting

d. Increase in blood pressure

Activity W *Think About It! Briefly answer the following question in the space provided.*

List four criteria that indicate that a person has recovered enough from the anesthesia to be transferred to the phase II section of the PACU.

_____

_____

_____

Activity X *Select the single best answer for each of the following questions.*

1. The use of TED stockings and performing leg exercises during phase II of recovery can help to prevent:

   a. Urinary retention

   b. Pneumonia

   c. Thrombus formation

   d. Wound infection

2. Assisting the patient to perform incentive spirometry after surgery can help to prevent:

   a. Wound infection

   b. Hemorrhage

   c. Constipation

   d. Pneumonia

Activity Y *Think About It! Briefly answer the following question in the space provided.*

List examples of topics the nurse will review with the patient and family members before the patient is discharged from the hospital or PACU.

_____

_____

_____

SUMMARY

Activity Z *Fill in the blanks using the words given in brackets.*

[anesthesia, air flow, sterile, pressure points, Aldrete, oxygenation]

1. The surgeon, surgical assistant, and scrub person are _____ team members.

2. _____ often leaves the patient unconscious or unable to feel or move parts of his body, leaving the patient totally dependent on the surgical team for safe care.

3. When a person has a/an _____ score of 7 or more, he is moved to phase II of recovery.

4. Monitoring the airway and _____ of a patient who is recovering from general anesthesia is very important in phase I of recovery.

5. Environmental controls within the restricted area, such as positive-pressure _____, help limit the patient's exposure to microbes.

6. Care is taken while positioning the patient for the surgical procedure to pad the _____.

Care of the Pediatric Patient

THE PEDIATRIC UNIT

Key Learning Point

■ Ways that a pediatric unit differs from an adult unit in an advanced care facility

Activity A *Think About It! Briefly answer the following question in the space provided.*

The pediatric unit at the hospital has arrangements for a family caregiver to stay overnight with the child in the hospital. This is called rooming-in. Why is rooming-in important for the child?

_____

_____

_____

EFFECTS OF HOSPITALIZATION ON THE CHILD AND FAMILY

Key Learning Point

■ The effects of hospitalization on the child and family

Activity B *Select the single best answer for the following question.*

1. Which of the following lists the stages a child may go through when separated from the caregiver?

   a. _____ Protest, despair, denial

   b. _____ Despair, disappointment, happiness

   c. _____ Denial, protest, playfulness

   d. _____ Protest, distress, joy

Activity C *The following are common reactions that children in a health care setting may exhibit when separated from a caregiver. Place a "P" next to reactions that depict the stage of protest and a "D" next to reactions that depict the stage of despair.*

1. _____ The child becomes depressed and listless.

2. _____ The child looks for the caregiver and keeps asking for him or her.

3. _____ The child thinks that the caregiver will not be coming back.

4. _____ The child cries and often refuses to be comforted by other people.

Activity D *Think About It! Briefly answer the following questions in the space provided.*

1. List ways that a family caregiver can participate in the care of a hospitalized child.

_____

_____

_____

2. How might a family caregiver behave because of the stress of having a hospitalized child?

_____

_____

_____

FEARS OF THE HOSPITALIZED CHILD

Key Learning Point

- Fears that hospitalized children commonly experience

Activity E *Think About It! Briefly answer the following questions in the space provided.*

1. A nursing assistant is helping a nurse administer an injection to a child. What explanation should be given to the child?

_____

_____

_____

2. A nursing assistant is caring for a child who needs daily dressing changes for the wound on his leg. The child is scared of the procedure and believes that he is being punished. What should the nursing assistant do?

_____

_____

_____

3. A young school-age child is being prepared for a tonsillectomy. What would be an appropriate explanation to give him regarding the surgical procedure?

_____

_____

_____

4. A nursing assistant is caring for a young child who is to be administered anesthesia in preparation for surgery. What would be an appropriate explanation regarding the process?

_____

_____

_____

THE IMPORTANCE OF PLAY

Key Learning Point

- The importance of play for children in an advanced care setting

Activity F *Place an "X" next to each correct answer for the following question.*

1. Which of the following are the advantages of play for the hospitalized child?

a. _____ Helps to relieve boredom

b. _____ Helps to minimize the stress of illness and hospitalization

c. _____ Helps the child to get discharged early

d. _____ Makes up for missed school time

e. _____ Allows the child to feel in charge and in control

Activity G *Fill in the blanks using the words given in brackets.*

[therapeutic, decrease, play]

1. The central activity area in the pediatric unit gives children the chance to _____ and socialize with each other.

2. _____ play is a technique that is often used to help a child have a better understanding of a treatment or surgical procedure.

3. Any type of play that increases the child's understanding of what is going to happen may help to _____ the child's anxiety.

PAIN AND THE PEDIATRIC PATIENT

Key Learning Points

- The different ways that children express pain
- The nursing assistant's role in helping to minimize a child's pain

Activity H *Think About It! Briefly answer the following questions in the space provided.*

1. List the ways that an infant may express pain.

2. List the ways that a toddler may express pain.

3. List the ways that an older child may express pain.

Activity I *Explain how children can use the FACES rating scale to identify their level of pain.*

Activity J *Think About It! Briefly answer the following question in the space provided.*

List some of the things a nursing assistant can do, in addition to reporting the pain to the nurse, when caring for a child who is in pain.

THE ROLE OF THE NURSING ASSISTANT IN CARING FOR PEDIATRIC PATIENTS

Key Learning Point

■ Some of the special considerations that a nursing assistant must take into account when providing basic nursing care for a pediatric patient

Activity K *Fill in the blanks using the words given in brackets.*

[appetite, increase, enteral, high, heal]

1. Children who are hospitalized need adequate nutrition in order to _____.

2. Being sick and in the hospital can further decrease a child's _____.

3. Offering small amounts of favorite foods that are _____ in nutritional value frequently throughout the day often results in a much greater intake of food.

4. Many sick children are also dehydrated and need to _____ their intake of fluids.

5. If a child is not able to take food or fluids orally for a period of time, _____ feedings might be provided through a nasogastric tube or a gastrostomy tube.

Activity L *Think About It! Briefly answer the following questions in the space provided.*

1. List ways that a child's urine output can be measured.

2. A nursing assistant is assisting a nurse perform venipuncture for a child. How can the nursing assistant help so the procedure is completed safely and accurately?

3. A child is restrained with the help of an elbow restraint to prevent him from pulling out his urinary catheter. What responsibilities does the nursing assistant have related to the restraint use?

_____

_____

_____

Activity M *Place an "X" next to each correct answer for the following question.*

1. Which of the following can be used for transporting young children?

a. _____ Wagons

b. _____ Bassinets

c. _____ Stretchers

d. _____ Strollers

e. _____ Small wheelchairs

COMMON DISORDERS AFFECTING CHILDREN

Key Learning Points

- The most common respiratory, cardiovascular, neurologic, gastrointestinal, endocrine, genitourinary, and musculoskeletal disorders that can affect children
- Special care needs of children with cancer

Activity N *Match the disorder given in Column A with its description given in Column B.*

Column A

_____ **1.** Congenital disorders

_____ **2.** Trauma

_____ **3.** Chronic illness

_____ **4.** Infectious diseases

Column B

a. Flare-ups and complications may lead to frequent hospitalizations.

b. Mostly results from accidents and often leads to death or disability.

c. These may cause dehydration or difficulty breathing.

d. These disorders are present at birth and may involve physical anomalies.

Activity O *Place an "X" next to each correct answer for the following question.*

1. A nursing assistant is caring for a child with a respiratory infection. Which of the following signs and symptoms in the child should be immediately reported to the nurse?

a. _____ Difficulty breathing

b. _____ Diarrhea

c. _____ Lips appear blue

d. _____ Change in the vital signs

e. _____ Loss of appetite

Activity P *Fill in the blanks using the words given in brackets.*

[lungs, respiratory syncytial virus, bronchioles, antibiotics, alveoli]

1. Bronchioles are the tiny airways that lead to the _____ in the lungs.

2. Pneumonia is the inflammation of the _____.

3. _____ is most common in children 6 months of age or younger and is rarely seen in healthy children older than age 2 years.

4. Respiratory syncytial virus (RSV) produces very thick mucus that quickly plugs the _____, making it difficult for the child to breathe.

5. _____ are not effective against RSV because it is caused by a virus.

Activity Q *Think About It! Briefly answer the following question in the space provided.*

A nursing assistant is caring for a child with respiratory syncytial virus. What are the responsibilities of the nursing assistant when caring for the child if the child is placed in a mist tent?

_____

_____

_____

Activity R *Select the single best answer for the following question.*

1. Which of the following body organs is affected by croup?
   a. Upper respiratory tract
   b. Brain
   c. Stomach
   d. Heart

Activity S *Fill in the blanks using the words given in brackets.*

[epiglottitis, humidified, croup, mist, oxygenation]

1. A child with _____ may have a harsh, bark-like cough and difficulty breathing.

2. Most types of croup are very effectively treated by using _____ air.

3. A pulse oximeter is used to monitor the child's _____ status.

4. A/An _____ tent may be used to provide extra humidity and oxygen.

5. _____ is a form of croup that is caused by *Haemophilus influenzae* type B, a type of bacteria.

Activity T *Place an "E" next to characteristics of epiglottitis and an "A" next to characteristics of asthma.*

1. _____ A form of croup

2. _____ Affects the bronchi and bronchioles

3. _____ Treated with inhaled medications called bronchodilators

4. _____ Caused by *Haemophilus influenzae* type B

5. _____ Causes inflammation of the epiglottis

6. _____ Caused by triggers such as allergies, activity, smoke, or weather changes

Activity U *Select the single best answer for each of the following questions.*

1. An acute asthma attack is usually treated with inhaled medications called _____.
   a. Antibiotics
   b. Analgesic
   c. Sedatives
   d. Bronchodilators

2. Which of the following conditions may be commonly seen in children who have asthma?
   a. Cardiovascular disease
   b. Respiratory infection
   c. Diarrhea
   d. Cancer

3. Which of the following is an inherited disorder that affects the body's exocrine glands?
   a. Cystic fibrosis
   b. Asthma
   c. Croup
   d. Epiglottitis

Activity V *Think About It! Briefly answer the following question in the space provided.*

How does cystic fibrosis affect a child?

_____

_____

_____

Activity W *Fill in the blanks using the words given in brackets.*

[anomaly, congenital, cyanotic, blood]

1. Most cardiovascular disorders in children are _____.

2. A physical _____ can be present in the structure of the heart, in the large blood vessels that carry blood from the heart, or both.

3. When there are multiple anomalies or the anomaly is severe, the heart is not able to send enough oxygen-rich _____ to the body's tissues.

4. An infant may become _____ because the tissues of the body are not receiving enough oxygen.

Activity X *Think About It! Briefly answer the following question in the space provided.*

A nursing assistant is caring for a child with a congenital cardiovascular anomaly. What are the responsibilities of the nursing assistant?

_____

_____

_____

Activity Y *Select the single best answer for each of the following questions.*

1. Which of the following is a common septal anomaly of the heart?

   a. Asthma

   b. Cystic fibrosis

   c. Patent foramen ovale

   d. Epiglottitis

2. When does the foramen ovale close in a healthy baby?

   a. Immediately after birth

   b. Within 24 hours of birth

   c. More than 1 week after birth

   d. More than 1 month after birth

Activity Z *Write down the correct sequence of blood circulation in the boxes provided below.*

1. Blood is pumped from the left atrium to the left ventricle.
2. Blood flows into the pulmonary vein.
3. Blood flows from the pulmonary artery to the lungs.
4. Blood is pumped from the right atrium to the right ventricle.
5. Blood is pumped out to the body.

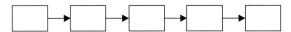

Activity AA *The figure below shows an opening between the two atria that is present during fetal development. Identify the opening and explain its significance.*

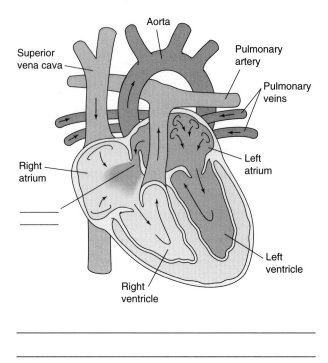

_____

_____

_____

Activity AB *Fill in the blanks using the words given in brackets.*

[aorta, lungs, coarctation, oxygenated, pulmonary]

1. In the developing fetus, a vessel called the ductus arteriosus connects the left pulmonary artery to the _____.

2. The ductus arteriosus lets _____ blood from the mother pass directly into the aorta, bypassing the baby's lungs.

3. After the baby is born and the heart begins to pump blood through the _____, the ductus arteriosus normally closes.

4. In a child with patent ductus arteriosus, the oxygenated blood flows from the aorta into the _____ artery, where it re-circulates through the lungs instead of going out to the body.

5. _____ of the aorta is a narrowing of the aorta shortly after it leaves the left ventricle.

Activity AC *Place an "X" next to each correct answer for the following questions.*

1. In tetralogy of Fallot, the child has four heart anomalies. Identify the anomalies among the following.

   a. _____ Narrowing of the pulmonary artery

   b. _____ A ventricular septal defect

   c. _____ An abnormally placed aorta that is positioned over a ventricular septal defect

   d. _____ Thickening of the muscular walls of the right ventricle

   e. _____ An atrial septal defect

   f. _____ An aortic aneurysm

2. Which of the following statements are true for transposition of the great arteries?

   a. _____ The right ventricle pumps oxygen-poor blood into the aorta.

   b. _____ The left ventricle pumps oxygen-rich blood into the pulmonary artery.

   c. _____ The pulmonary artery and aorta are switched.

   d. _____ The oxygen-rich blood is pumped to the whole body.

   e. _____ The oxygen-poor blood is pumped into the lungs.

Activity AD *Place a "C" next to characteristics of cerebral palsy, an "H" next to characteristics of hydrocephalus, and an "S" next to characteristics of spina bifida.*

1. _____ It is caused by damage to the cerebrum, the part of the brain involved with motor control.

2. _____ It results from a build-up of cerebrospinal fluid.

3. _____ It is a congenital anomaly of the vertebrae.

4. _____ To relieve the pressure, a shunt may be placed to drain the fluid, relieving the cerebrospinal fluid pressure.

5. _____ The vertebrae do not close properly during development, leaving the spinal cord exposed.

Activity AE *Fill in the blanks using the words given in brackets.*

[viral, bacterial, meninges]

1. The three layers of connective tissue that surround the brain and spinal cord are called

   _____.

2. _____ meningitis is most common in people older than age 16 years.

3. _____ meningitis may occur quite suddenly after an upper respiratory tract infection.

Activity AF *Place an "X" next to each correct answer for the following question.*

1. Which of the following are the most common symptoms of meningitis?

   a. _____ Fever

   b. _____ Irritability

   c. _____ Diarrhea

   d. _____ Stiff neck

   e. _____ Cough

Activity AG *Identify the procedure shown in the figure. What is the purpose of this procedure?*

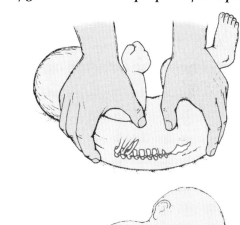
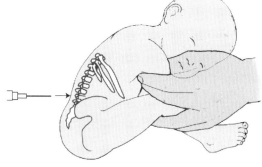

_____

_____

_____

Activity AH *Place an "X" next to each correct answer for the following question.*

1. Which of the following should be closely monitored when caring for a child with meningitis?

   a. _____ Decrease in blood pressure

   b. _____ Food preferences

   c. _____ Change in level of consciousness

   d. _____ Intake and output of fluids

   e. _____ Increase in irritability

Activity AI *Think About It! Briefly answer the following question in the space provided.*

List some common causes of traumatic brain injury (TBI) and spinal cord injury in children.

_____

_____

_____

Activity AJ *Fill in the blanks using the words given in brackets.*

[dehydration, appendicitis, bowels, rotavirus]

1. Inflammation or infection of the appendix is

   called _____.

2. Diarrhea, vomiting, or both in a small child

   can quickly lead to _____.

3. The most common cause of severe diarrhea and vomiting in infants and children younger

   than age 5 years is _____ infection.

4. Rotavirus is a virus that infects the

   _____.

Activity AK *Place an "X" next to each correct answer for the following question.*

1. What precautions should a nursing assistant take to prevent the spread of infection when caring for a child who has infectious diarrhea?

   a. _____ Wash the hands carefully and frequently.

   b. _____ Ensure that the child has a full meal.

   c. _____ Keep the child away from family members and other patients.

   d. _____ Wear gloves and a gown when changing diapers.

   e. _____ Practice safe disposal of diapers, clothing, and linens soiled with feces.

Activity AL *Think About It! Briefly answer the following question in the space provided.*

What are the responsibilities of the nursing assistant when taking care of a child with diarrhea?

_____

_____

_____

Activity AM *Identify the disorder shown in the figure.*

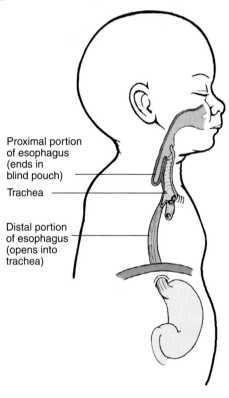

Proximal portion of esophagus (ends in blind pouch)

Trachea

Distal portion of esophagus (opens into trachea)

_____

Activity AN *Identify the disorder shown in the figure.*

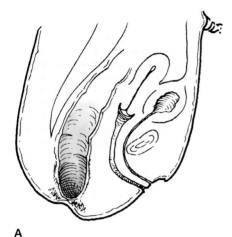

A

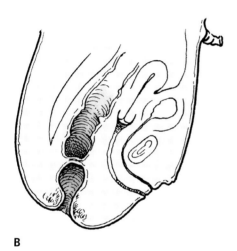

B

_____

Activity AO *Place a "U" next to characteristics of umbilical hernias, an "I" next to characteristics of inguinal hernias, and an "H" next to characteristics of hiatal hernias.*

1. _____ Occurs when a loop of intestine bulges through the abdominal wall in the groin area.

2. _____ Occurs when a loop of intestine bulges through the abdominal wall near the umbilicus.

3. _____ May push the heart to the right side and squeeze the left lung, causing severe difficulty with breathing.

4. _____ Usually surgically repaired soon after they are discovered because they can become strangulated.

5. _____ Usually close by themselves by the time the child is 3 years old.

6. _____ Occurs when the abdominal organs pass through the opening in the diaphragm that allows the esophagus to pass into the abdominal cavity.

Activity AP *Fill in the blanks using the words given in brackets.*

[peritonitis, right, appendix, omphalocele, appendectomy]

1. In _____, the infant's intestines or other abdominal organs protrude through an opening around the umbilicus.

2. The _____ is a tiny, closed pouch that dangles from the end of the cecum.

3. Signs of appendicitis include fever, nausea and vomiting, and _____ lower quadrant abdominal pain.

4. _____ is the inflammation of the thin membrane that lines the abdominal wall and the organs in the abdominal cavity.

5. Appendicitis is treated by surgical removal of the appendix, called a/an _____.

Activity AQ *Think About It! Briefly answer the following question in the space provided.*

What are the responsibilities of the nursing assistant when taking care of a child who has undergone an appendectomy?

_____

_____

_____

Activity AR *Select the single best answer for each of the following questions.*

1. Type 1 diabetes mellitus is caused by destruction of the insulin-producing cells of the _____.
   a. Brain
   b. Liver
   c. Stomach
   d. Pancreas

2. Which of the following is usually one of the first signs of type 1 diabetes mellitus?

   a. Weight gain

   b. Hyperactivity

   c. Slowed growth

   d. Headache

Activity AS *Place an "X" next to each correct answer for the following questions.*

1. Which of the following factors must be balanced to maintain blood sugar?

   a. _____ Water intake

   b. _____ Energy expenditures

   c. _____ Food intake

   d. _____ Sleep

   e. _____ Insulin

2. Which of the following can cause hypoglycemia?

   a. _____ Delayed meal

   b. _____ Too much sleep

   c. _____ Not enough food

   d. _____ Too much insulin

   e. _____ Too little exercise

Activity AT *Think About It! Briefly answer the following questions in the space provided.*

1. What are the responsibilities of the nursing assistant when caring for a child with type 1 diabetes mellitus?

2. List the signs and symptoms of hypoglycemia that should be reported to the nurse immediately.

Activity AU *Fill in the blanks using the words given in brackets.*

[cryptorchidism, epispadias, hypospadias, genitourinary]

1. _____ is a term used to describe the urinary and reproductive systems together.

2. _____ occurs when a baby boy's testes fail to descend.

3. When the urethral opening is located on the underside of the penis, instead of on the tip, it is known as _____.

4. When the urethral opening is located on the top of the penis, it is known as _____.

Activity AV *Place an "X" next to each correct answer for the following question.*

1. Which of the following methods are commonly used to treat fractures?

   a. _____ Open reduction

   b. _____ Closed reduction

   c. _____ Internal fixation

   d. _____ Application of a soft bandage

   e. _____ Heat application

Activity AW *Think About It! Briefly answer the following questions in the space provided.*

1. What are the responsibilities of the nursing assistant when caring for a child who has a cast?

2. List the signs or symptoms that should be immediately reported to the nurse when taking care of a child who has a cast.

Activity AX *Fill in the blanks using the words given in brackets.*

[autoimmune, systemic, joint, splints, arthritis]

1. _____ is an inflammation of the joints that is usually associated with pain and stiffness.

2. In a/an _____ disorder, the body's immune system begins to attack the body's own tissues.

3. _____ juvenile rheumatoid arthritis can affect other organs, such as the heart, lungs, and liver, as well as the joints.

4. Medications, physical therapy, and surgery are all used to maintain mobility and preserve _____ function.

5. Range-of motion-exercises, heat application, and the use of _____ are all necessary parts of daily physical therapy for juvenile rheumatoid arthritis.

Activity AY *Match the term given in Column A with its appropriate description given in Column B.*

Column A

_____ 1. Muscular dystrophy

_____ 2. Leukemia

_____ 3. Leukocytes

_____ 4. Lymphomas

_____ 5. Nephroblastoma

Column B

a. Cancers of the lymphatic system

b. A group of inherited disorders that cause the skeletal muscles to become progressively weaker over time

c. Cancer of the kidney

d. Cancer of the blood-forming cells in the bone marrow

e. White blood cells

Activity AZ *Think About It! Briefly answer the following questions in the space provided.*

1. Angelina, a 5-year-old girl who has been diagnosed with leukemia, has to undergo bone marrow transplantation. How are children usually prepared for the transplant?

_____

_____

_____

2. The child may be placed in reverse isolation because she is at high risk for becoming very ill if she gets an infectious disease. What precautions should be taken when caring for the child in reverse isolation?

_____

_____

_____

CHILD ABUSE

Key Learning Point

■ Signs of child abuse and the nursing assistant's role in reporting suspected abuse

Activity BA *Think About It! Briefly answer the following question in the space provided.*

1. What are the responsibilities of a nursing assistant when he suspects that a child has been abused?

_____

_____

_____

SUMMARY

Activity BB *Fill in the blanks using the words given in brackets.*

[boredom, pediatric, stressful, FACES, therapeutic]

1. _____ units are designed especially for children and their families.

2. A child's illness or injury and hospitalization is _____ for both the child and family.

3. Play and other activities are important to help relieve _____ and stress.

4. _____ play can be used to help a child have a better understanding of a treatment or surgical procedure, which helps to decrease anxiety.

5. The _____ pain rating scale is a useful tool that can help a young child express the level of pain she is experiencing.

Activity BC *Match the disorders given in Column A with the organ systems they affect in Column B.*

Column A

_____ 1. Appendicitis

_____ 2. Muscular dystrophy

_____ 3. Cryptorchidism

_____ 4. Type 1 diabetes mellitus

_____ 5. Meningitis

_____ 6. Patent ductus arteriosus

_____ 7. Croup

Column B

a. Neurologic

b. Gastrointestinal

c. Endocrine

d. Genitourinary

e. Musculoskeletal

f. Respiratory

g. Cardiovascular

CHAPTER 12

Care of the Obstetric Patient

HIGH-RISK PREGNANCY

Key Learning Points

- Common pre-existing health conditions that can complicate pregnancy
- Some of the complications that can develop during pregnancy
- Multiple gestations as a cause of high-risk pregnancy

Activity A *Think About It! Briefly answer the following questions in the space provided.*

1. What is meant by the term "high-risk pregnancy"?

   _____

   _____

   _____

2. List three complications that can occur as the result of high blood glucose levels in a diabetic pregnant patient.

   _____

   _____

   _____

3. How can heart diseases complicate a pregnancy?

   _____

   _____

   _____

Activity B *Place an "X" next to each correct answer for the following questions.*

1. Which of the following interventions may be used to help reduce the strain on the mother's heart during the pregnancy?

   a. _____ Frequent monitoring

   b. _____ Medication

   c. _____ High protein diet

   d. _____ Increased fluid intake

   e. _____ Bed rest

2. Which of the following side effects may result from the use of illegal drugs, alcohol, and tobacco during pregnancy?

   a. _____ Excessive birth weight

   b. _____ Congenital anomalies

   c. _____ Mental retardation

   d. _____ Growth retardation

   e. _____ Urinary tract infection

Activity C *Identify the type of pregnancy shown in the given figure. How does it occur?*

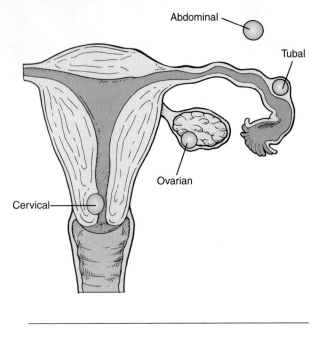

Abdominal

Tubal

Ovarian

Cervical

_____

_____

_____

Activity D *Select the single best answer for each of the following questions.*

1. Which one of the following sites is the most common location of an ectopic pregnancy?

   a. Abdomen

   b. Fallopian tube

   c. Ovary

   d. Cervix

2. The fertilized egg moves through the fallopian tube into the uterus and attaches itself to the endometrium. This process is called _____.

   a. Transformation

   b. Transplantation

   c. Implantation

   d. Adhesion

Activity E *Match the terms given in Column A with their descriptions given in Column B.*

Column A

_____ 1. Threatened abortion

_____ 2. Spontaneous abortion

_____ 3. Complete abortion

_____ 4. Missed abortion

_____ 5. Incomplete abortion

Column B

a. All of the products of conception are expelled.

b. Some, but not all, of the products of conception are expelled.

c. The loss of the fetus before the 20th week of pregnancy.

d. Cramping and bleeding are experienced, which may indicate impending spontaneous abortion.

e. The fetus dies and the products of conception remain in the uterus.

Activity F *Think About It! Briefly answer the following questions in the space provided.*

1. List responsibilities that the nursing assistant may have when caring for the patient who is having a spontaneous abortion.

   _____

   _____

   _____

2. A nursing assistant is caring for a patient with an incompetent cervix who is in the sixth month of pregnancy. The patient is on complete bed rest in preparation for a cervical cerclage procedure. What is an incompetent cervix?

   _____

   _____

   _____

Activity G *Select the single best answer for the following question.*

1. If dilation of the cervix is detected in the early stages of pregnancy, which of the following procedures may be performed by the doctor?
   a. Cesarean section
   b. Shirodkar procedure
   c. Hysterectomy
   d. Tubectomy

Activity H *Place an "X" next to each correct answer for the following question.*

1. Which of the following signs and symptoms should be immediately reported to the nurse when caring for a patient with incompetent cervix?
   a. _____ Abdominal pain
   b. _____ Nausea
   c. _____ Fluid leaking from the vagina
   d. _____ Increased respiratory rate
   e. _____ Uterine contractions

Activity I *Select the single best answer for the following question.*

1. Which of the following symptoms is prominent in patients experiencing hyperemesis gravidarum?
   a. Headache
   b. Urinary urgency
   c. Fluid leaking from the vagina
   d. Nausea and vomiting

Activity J *Think About It! Briefly answer the following question in the space provided.*

What are the special concerns when caring for a patient with hyperemesis gravidarum? List the nursing assistant's responsibilities.

_____
_____
_____

Activity K *Select the single best answer for the following question.*

1. Which of the following blood pressure values may indicate the presence of gestational hypertension in a pregnant woman?
   a. 110/60 mm Hg
   b. 130/80 mm Hg
   c. 120/70 mm Hg
   d. 150/100 mm Hg

Activity L *Think About It! Briefly answer the following question in the space provided.*

List the observations that should be immediately reported to the nurse when caring for a patient with gestational hypertension.

_____
_____
_____

Activity M *Fill in the blanks using the words given in brackets.*

[oxygen, placenta, upper, second]

1. Gestational diabetes develops during the _____ trimester of pregnancy in a woman who has never had diabetes before.
2. The _____ is an organ that develops along with the fetus.
3. One of the main roles of the placenta is to transfer _____ and nutrients from the mother's blood to the fetus' blood.
4. Normally, the placenta attaches in the _____ portion of the uterus.

Activity N *Select the single best answer for the following question.*

1. In placenta previa, the placenta attaches in the _____.
   a. Upper portion of uterus
   b. Lower portion of uterus
   c. Middle portion of uterus
   d. Upper portion of vagina

Activity O *Think About It! Briefly answer the following questions in the space provided.*

1. A nursing assistant is caring for a patient who had placenta previa and who has undergone caesarean delivery. How could placenta previa have affected her baby?

   _____

   _____

   _____

2. Why does the patient with placenta previa have an increased risk of hemorrhage after delivery?

   _____

   _____

   _____

Activity P *Place an "X" next to each correct answer for the following question.*

1. Which of the following may be signs of worsening abruptio placentae?

   a. _____ Abdominal pain

   b. _____ A firm uterus

   c. _____ Tachycardia

   d. _____ Hypertension

   e. _____ Vomiting

Activity Q *Select the single best answer for the following question.*

1. Pre-term labor begins _____.

   a. Before the 20th week of pregnancy

   b. Between the 20th week and the 37th week of pregnancy

   c. After the 37th week of pregnancy

   d. Before the 12th week of pregnancy

Activity R *Think About It! Briefly answer the following questions in the space provided.*

1. List the risk factors for pre-term labor.

   _____

   _____

   _____

2. What observations should be immediately reported to the nurse when caring for a patient with pre-term labor?

   _____

   _____

   _____

Activity S *Select the single best answer for the following question.*

1. In which period of gestation does the pre-term premature rupture of membranes occur?

   a. Just before the pregnancy due date

   b. Before the 37th week of pregnancy

   c. After the 37th week of pregnancy

   d. After the 20th week of pregnancy

Activity T *Think About It! Briefly answer the following question in the space provided.*

What are the responsibilities of a nursing assistant when caring for a patient with pre-term premature rupture of membranes?

   _____

   _____

   _____

Activity U *Select the single best answer for the following question.*

1. Which of the following occurs when one egg is fertilized by one sperm and then divides into two separate fetuses?

   a. Monozygotic twins

   b. Fraternal twins

   c. Dizygotic twins

   d. Conjoined twins

LABOR AND DELIVERY

Key Learning Points

- The stages of labor and a vaginal delivery and the responsibilities of a nursing assistant during each stage
- Reasons why a cesarean delivery might be necessary and the responsibilities a nursing assistant may have during a cesarean delivery

Activity V *Think About It! Briefly answer the following question in the space provided.*

List the responsibilities of a nursing assistant when caring for a patient after a vaginal delivery.

_____

_____

_____

Activity W *Select the single best answer for each of the following questions.*

1. A registered nurse who completes 1 to 2 years of additional graduate training to learn how to assist a woman through pregnancy and childbirth is known as a/an _____.
   a. Nurse midwife
   b. Obstetrician
   c. Head nurse
   d. Nurse anesthetist

2. As pregnancy progresses, changes occur in the woman's body in preparation for labor and the delivery of the baby. Which of the following signs may indicate that labor will begin within the next 2 weeks?
   a. Bloody show
   b. Braxton Hicks contractions
   c. Lightening
   d. Bulging around the perineal area

Activity X *Fill in the blanks using the words given in brackets.*

[irregular, bloody, primipara, multipara, regular]

1. _____ show is a blood-tinged vaginal discharge that may appear to be mixed with a large amount of thick mucus.

2. Braxton Hicks contractions are _____ contractions of the uterus that occur throughout pregnancy but may occur with more frequency as labor approaches.

3. The first stage of labor begins with the onset of the first _____ contractions and ends when the cervix is fully dilated.

4. A woman delivering her first baby is called a/an _____.

5. A/an _____ is a woman who has delivered a baby before.

Activity Y *Select the single best answer for each of the following questions.*

1. For a primipara, the first stage of labor lasts an average of _____.
   a. 6 to 8 hours
   b. 10 to 12 hours
   c. 12 to 24 hours
   d. 24 to 36 hours

2. For a multipara, the first stage of labor lasts an average of _____.
   a. 6 to 8 hours
   b. 10 to 12 hours
   c. 8 to 12 hours
   d. 8 to 10 hours

Activity Z *Place a "T" next to characteristics of true labor and an "F" next to characteristics of false labor.*

1. _____ The amniotic sac remains intact.

2. _____ Walking may cause the contractions to become stronger.

3. _____ Contractions become regular, longer, and more frequent as labor progresses.

4. _____ Walking may cause the contractions to decrease or go away.

5. _____ The amniotic sac may rupture.

6. _____ The cervix remains closed.

7. _____ The contractions remain irregular and short.

8. _____ The cervix progressively dilates.

Activity AA *Following are the characteristics of the stages of labor. Place an "E" next to characteristics of early phase, an "M" next to characteristics of mid phase of labor, and a "T" next to characteristics of transitional phase of labor.*

1. _____ Contractions occur 5 to 8 minutes apart, lasting 20 to 35 seconds each.

2. _____ The cervix is dilated 4 to 7 cm.

3. ____ Contractions occur 3 to 5 minutes apart, and each may last for 40 to 60 seconds.

4. ____ The cervix dilates from 7 to 10 cm.

5. ____ The cervix is dilated 0 to 3 cm.

6. ____ Contractions occur every 2 to 3 minutes, and each can last for as long as 80 seconds.

Activity AB *Select the single best answer for each of the following questions.*

1. At which stage of labor does crowning occur?
   a. Early latent phase
   b. Active phase
   c. Transitional phase
   d. Second stage of labor

2. The second stage of labor lasts an average of _____.
   a. 10 minutes
   b. 20 to 50 minutes
   c. 1 hour
   d. 2 hours

Activity AC *Select the single best answer for the following question.*

1. A woman is considered to be hemorrhaging if the perineal pad is completely soaked within _____.
   a. 1 hour
   b. 2 hours
   c. 3 hours
   d. 4 hours

Activity AD *Think About It! Briefly answer the following question in the space provided.*

What special considerations are necessary when assisting a new mother with urination immediately after a vaginal delivery?

_____

_____

_____

Activity AE *Place an "X" next to each correct answer for the following question.*

1. Which of the following conditions might make a scheduled cesarean section necessary?
   a. ____ Preterm labor
   b. ____ Abruptio placentae
   c. ____ Cephalopelvic disproportion
   d. ____ Breech presentation
   e. ____ Shoulder presentation

Activity AF *Match the terms given in Column A with their descriptions given in Column B.*

Column A
____ **1.** Uterine rupture
____ **2.** Breech presentation
____ **3.** Dystocia
____ **4.** Prolapsed cord
____ **5.** Nuchal cord

Column B
a. Labor that is long and difficult and does not progress normally
b. The umbilical cord is looped one or more times around the baby's neck
c. A loop of umbilical cord slips past the presenting part of the baby, through the cervix, and into the vagina
d. Legs or buttocks as presenting parts of the baby
e. The uterus rips open, often resulting in the death of the baby

Activity AG *Think About It! Briefly answer the following question in the space provided.*

In addition to the routine postpartum care, what postoperative care should be provided to a patient who has had a cesarean section?

_____

_____

_____

POSTPARTUM COMPLICATIONS

Key Learning Point

■ Common postpartum complications and observations that the nursing assistant should immediately report to the nurse

Activity AH *Place an "X" next to each correct answer for the following question.*

1. Which of the following are common postpartum complications?
   a. _____ Hemorrhage
   b. _____ Gastroenteritis
   c. _____ Pressure ulcers
   d. _____ Infection
   e. _____ Thrombophlebitis

Activity AI *Fill in the blanks using the words given in brackets.*

[superficial, puerperal, thrombophlebitis, placenta]

1. Late postpartum hemorrhage may be caused by fragments of the _____ left behind in the uterus or by an infection.

2. _____ infection is an infection that develops after childbirth.

3. _____ is inflammation of the lining of a blood vessel, usually a vein, caused by a blood clot.

4. _____ thrombophlebitis affects the veins near the surface of the legs, causing redness and pain.

Activity AJ *Select the single best answer for each of the following questions.*

1. Which of the following signs may indicate a puerperal infection in a new mother?
   a. Chills
   b. Bleeding
   c. Abdominal pain
   d. Edema

2. Which of the following complications may cause a pulmonary embolism?
   a. Hemorrhage
   b. Superficial thrombophlebitis
   c. Puerperal infection
   d. Deep vein thrombophlebitis

Activity AK *Think About It! Briefly answer the following question in the space provided.*

What special considerations should the nursing assistant keep in mind when providing care for a patient who has postpartum thrombophlebitis?

_____

_____

_____

SUMMARY

Activity AL *Fill in the blanks using the words given in brackets.*

[labor, spontaneous, late, ectopic, second]

1. A/an _____ pregnancy occurs when a fertilized egg implants outside of the uterus.

2. A/An _____ abortion results in the loss of the fetus before the 20th week of pregnancy.

3. _____ is the process during which the woman's uterus contracts and expels the baby.

4. The _____ stage of labor begins with the complete dilation of the cervix and ends with the birth of the baby.

5. A/An _____ postpartum hemorrhage can occur up to 6 weeks after delivery.

CHAPTER 13

Care of the Psychiatric Patient

SETTINGS FOR PSYCHIATRIC CARE

Key Learning Point

- Settings where psychiatric care may be provided

Activity A *Fill in the blanks using the words given in brackets.*

[residential, mental, rehabilitation, outpatient]

1. Psychiatric patients are people who are receiving health care for a/an _____ illness.

2. _____ mental health clinics offer services such as counseling, medication, and support groups that help the person to manage the disorder while remaining in the community.

3. Long-term psychiatric care facilities are _____ facilities for people who cannot function on their own as the result of their mental illness.

4. The focus of psychiatric _____ is to help the person manage her disorder, obtain the skills she needs to live in the community, and function at her highest possible level.

Activity B *Select the single best answer for the following question.*

1. Which of the following psychiatric care settings provides care to people who are experiencing mental crises that may cause them to harm themselves or others?
   - a. Long-term psychiatric care facilities
   - b. Outpatient mental health clinics
   - c. Acute psychiatric care facilities
   - d. Psychiatric rehabilitation facilities

THE NURSING ASSISTANT'S ROLE IN PROVIDING PSYCHIATRIC CARE

Key Learning Point

- Responsibilities of a nursing assistant who works in a psychiatric care setting

Activity C *Match the job titles of health care workers who specialize in psychiatric care given in Column A with their descriptions given in Column B.*

Column A	Column B
____ 1. Psychiatrist	a. An unlicensed health care worker who may or may not be certified as a nursing assistant
____ 2. Psychiatric clinical nurse specialist	

_____ **3.** Psychiatric nurse

_____ **4.** Psychiatric aide

_____ **5.** Psychologist

b. A person with a doctoral degree in clinical psychology who provides counseling services

c. A registered nurse who has obtained additional training in psychiatric–mental health nursing

d. A medical doctor trained in diagnosing and treating mental illness who serves as the leader of the psychiatric health care team

e. A registered nurse who has obtained a master's degree in psychiatric–mental health nursing

Activity D *Select the single best answer for the following question.*

1. Patients learn about self-care topics, such as hand washing and personal hygiene, in which one of the following groups?

  a. Psycho-educational groups

  b. Activities of daily living (ADL) groups

  c. Social skill-building groups

  d. Recreational groups

Activity E *Think About It! Briefly answer the following question in the space provided.*

List the benefits of a therapeutic environment.

_____

_____

_____

THERAPEUTIC COMMUNICATION

Key Learning Point

■ Goals of therapeutic communication and some common therapeutic communication techniques

Activity F *Match the therapeutic communication techniques given in Column A with their uses given in Column B.*

Column A

_____ **1.** Broad opening

_____ **2.** Encouraging

_____ **3.** Redirecting

_____ **4.** Clarifying

_____ **5.** Interpreting

Column B

a. Helps to prevent misunderstandings

b. Helps to reveal patient concerns

c. Invites the patient to talk

d. Returns the focus of the conversation to the patient

e. Invites the patient to continue talking

Activity G *Think About It! Briefly answer the following question in the space provided.*

A nursing assistant is caring for a patient with a psychiatric disorder. How can the nursing assistant improve communication with the patient?

_____

_____

_____

Activity H *Select the single best answer for each of the following questions.*

1. A nursing assistant finds that a patient spends a lot of time flattering him, saying he is very kind and efficient. What should the nursing assistant do?

  a. Redirect the conversation.

  b. Encourage the conversation.

  c. Stop the conversation.

  d. Scold the patient.

2. A nursing assistant is caring for a patient with psychiatric disorder. Which of the following should he do when he does not understand what the patient is telling him?

  a. Agree with the patient to be polite.

  b. Jot down the statements and ask the nurse for clarification.

  c. Ignore the patient.

  d. Ask the patient to clarify.

WORKPLACE SAFETY

Key Learning Points

- Measures to ensure safety in the workplace
- Conditions that may make restraint or seclusion necessary
- The nursing assistant's role in caring for a patient who has been restrained or who is in seclusion

Activity I *Fill in the blanks using the words given in brackets.*

[overstimulating, restraint, seclusion]

1. If a patient behaves in a way that poses a risk to himself or others, the doctor may order the use of a/an _____.

2. _____ involves placing the person alone in a specially equipped locked room.

3. The goal of seclusion is to limit the patient's exposure to people or situations that are

   _____.

Activity J *Place an "X" next to each correct answer for the following questions.*

1. Which of the following items are commonly prohibited in psychiatric units?
   a. _____ Books
   b. _____ Plastic water pitcher
   c. _____ Perfume bottles
   d. _____ Clothes hangers
   e. _____ Fingernail clippers

2. Which of the following statements are true regarding the use of restraints and seclusion for a mentally ill patient?
   a. _____ They are ordered by the doctor.
   b. _____ They are only used when a patient poses a threat to herself or others.
   c. _____ They are used as punishment.
   d. _____ When used, the patient must be monitored at least every 15 minutes.
   e. _____ They are for long-term use.

TREATMENT OF PSYCHIATRIC DISORDERS

Key Learning Points

- Four main categories of medications used to treat psychiatric disorders
- Observations a nursing assistant may make that should be reported to the nurse when caring for a patient who is being treated with medication for a psychiatric disorder
- Psychotherapy to help a person with a psychiatric disorder
- The nursing assistant's role in caring for a patient who is receiving electroconvulsive therapy

Activity K *Fill in the blanks using the words given in brackets.*

[synapse, excitatory, antidepressants, reuptake, inhibitory, neurotransmitters]

1. _____ are medications used to treat clinical depression.

2. Antidepressants work by affecting certain _____ in the brain.

3. A/An _____ is the gap between the axon of one neuron and the dendrites of the next.

4. _____ neurotransmitters cause an action to happen.

5. _____ neurotransmitters stop an action from happening.

6. The process during which a neurotransmitter is released, causes an action, and returns to the axon to be stored for later use is called

   _____.

Activity L *Select the single best answer for each of the following questions.*

1. Which of the following antidepressants is rarely used because of potential fatal side effects?
   a. Monoamine oxidase inhibitors
   b. Benzodiazepines
   c. Antipsychotics
   d. Mood stabilizers

2. If a patient undergoing antidepressant therapy experiences sleepiness or insomnia, which of the following measures may help him overcome the complication?

   a. Stopping the medication immediately

   b. Changing the type of medication

   c. Decreasing the dosage of medication

   d. Changing the time the medication is taken

3. How long does it usually take for an antidepressant to become effective after a person starts taking it?

   a. 1 week

   b. 2 to 4 weeks

   c. 3 to 6 weeks

   d. 5 weeks

4. Which of the following side effects may be observed in patients taking benzodiazepines?

   a. Constipation

   b. Urinary retention

   c. Dry mouth

   d. Physical dependence

5. Which of the following medications may be used in the treatment of bipolar disorder?

   a. Valium

   b. Buspirone

   c. Lithium

   d. Amitriptyline

Activity M *Think About It! Briefly answer the following questions in the space provided.*

1. Explain what bipolar disorder is.

   _____

   _____

   _____

2. How does a mood stabilizer work to help a patient with bipolar disorder?

   _____

   _____

   _____

Activity N *Fill in the blanks using the words given in brackets.*

[hallucinations, manic, extrapyramidal, antipsychotics]

1. _____ are medications used to treat psychotic disorders, such as schizophrenia.

2. A person with a psychotic disorder may have delusions and _____.

3. Antipsychotics may be used to treat the _____ phase of bipolar disorder.

4. Antipsychotics can cause very serious and potentially life-threatening neurologic side effects, called _____ side effects.

Activity O *Match the side effects of medications used to treat psychotic disorders given in Column A with their descriptions given in Column B.*

Column A	Column B
_____ 1. Dystonia	a. Involuntary movement of the muscles of the head, neck, and extremities
_____ 2. Akathisia	
_____ 3. Drug-induced Parkinsonism	b. The development of a shuffling gait, a stooped posture, drooling, and tremors
_____ 4. Tardive dyskinesia	c. An intense feeling of restlessness during which the person cannot sit still
	d. Acute muscle spasms or stiffness in the neck, back, or body that may affect the person's ability to breathe and swallow

Activity P *Think About It! Briefly answer the following question in the space provided.*

What are the primary responsibilities of a nursing assistant when caring for a patient taking antipsychotic medications?

_____

_____

_____

Activity Q *Given below are descriptions related to psychotherapy and electroconvulsive therapy. Place a "P" next to the descriptions belonging to psychotherapy and an "E" next to the descriptions belonging to electroconvulsive therapy.*

1. _____ An electrical shock is delivered to the patient's brain through electrodes applied to the scalp.

2. _____ It helps the person to explore feelings, attitudes, thinking, and behavior.

3. _____ It helps the patient to gain a better understanding of herself and to make positive changes in her life.

4. _____ It is used to treat severe depression that does not respond to other types of treatment.

5. _____ During the procedure, the person is given oxygen and may be assisted with breathing if necessary.

6. _____ Patients are administered an anesthetic and a muscle relaxant before the therapy.

Activity R *Think About It! Briefly answer the following question in the space provided.*

What are the responsibilities of a nursing assistant when preparing a patient for electroconvulsive therapy?

_____

_____

_____

CARING FOR PATIENTS WITH SPECIFIC PSYCHIATRIC DISORDERS

Key Learning Point

- Some of the more common psychiatric disorders and the special considerations a nursing assistant should be aware of when caring for patients with these disorders

Activity S *Select the single best answer for the following question.*

1. In which one of the following psychiatric disorders might the person be unable to speak and feel like running away?
   a. Obsessive-compulsive disorder
   b. Bipolar disorder
   c. Panic disorder
   d. Post-traumatic stress disorder

Activity T *Fill in the blanks using the words given in brackets.*

[psychotherapy, anxiolytic, obsessions, phobia]

1. Recurrent unwanted thoughts are known as

   _____.

2. A person with a/an _____ has an excessive, abnormal fear of an object or situation.

3. Benzodiazepines are a class of _____ drugs commonly used to treat anxiety disorders.

4. _____ focuses on helping the person to learn new ways of coping by teaching the person to rethink his response to a situation.

Activity U *Select the single best answer for the following question.*

1. Which of the following tactics can a nursing assistant use to help lower the anxiety level of a patient with an anxiety disorder?
   a. Remain calm and speak in a reassuring manner.
   b. Use a bossy or demanding tone of voice.
   c. Threaten to take back liberties given to the patient.
   d. Insist that the patient is incorrect.

Activity V *Fill in the blanks using the words given in brackets.*

[suicidal, psychotic, clinical, bipolar, lithium]

1. _____ depression is a disorder characterized by intense feelings of sadness and hopelessness that do not go away, even with time.

2. _____ depression is a very severe clinical depression that causes the person to lose contact with reality.

3. A person with depression may have difficulty thinking or making decisions, feelings of guilt and worthlessness, and _____ ideation.

4. _____ is most commonly used to keep the person's mood somewhere in between the two extremes.

5. _____ disorder is a mental health disorder that causes the person to have mood swings.

Activity W *Think About It! Briefly answer the following question in the space provided.*

List the signs or symptoms that may indicate lithium toxicity that the nursing assistant should report to the nurse right away.

_____

_____

_____

Activity X *Select the single best answer for each of the following questions.*

1. Which of the following may be a sign of schizophrenia?
   a. Obsession
   b. Delusions
   c. Mania
   d. Headache

2. Which of the following abnormalities is usually found in people with schizophrenia?
   a. High lithium levels
   b. Decreased fluid levels
   c. Less brain tissue
   d. Low sodium levels

Activity Y *Fill in the blanks using the words given in brackets.*

[paranoid, affect, inappropriate, antipsychotic, cluster A, cluster B, cluster C, polydipsia]

1. _____ is a person's facial expression.

2. A person with schizophrenia may have _____ affect, which means that the person's facial expression does not match the situation.

3. People with schizophrenia will have fluid restrictions if they have _____.

4. Many people with schizophrenia are _____, which means they are suspicious and distrustful of others.

5. Schizophrenia can usually be controlled with _____ medication.

6. _____ personality disorders are defined by odd or eccentric behavior.

7. _____ personality disorders are defined by dramatic, unpredictable, and emotional behavior.

8. _____ personality disorders are defined by fearful or shy behavior.

Activity Z *Think About It! Briefly answer the following question in the space provided.*

List a few traits found in most people with personality disorders.

_____

_____

_____

Activity AA *Place an "X" next to each correct answer for the following question.*

1. Which of the following indicates withdrawal symptoms when use of a particular abused substance is discontinued?
   a. _____ Tremors
   b. _____ Hypotension
   c. _____ Nausea and vomiting
   d. _____ Decreased heart rate
   e. _____ Anxiety

Activity AB *Think About It! Briefly answer the following question in the space provided.*

What are the responsibilities of a nursing assistant caring for a patient with an eating disorder?

_____

_____

_____

SUMMARY

Activity AC *Fill in the blanks using the words given in brackets.*

[electroconvulsive, withdrawal, neurologic, schizophrenia, communication]

1. When caring for a patient who is taking an antipsychotic medication, it is important to watch the person carefully for _____ side effects.

2. A person with a substance abuse disorder may go through _____ when use of the substance is discontinued.

3. Good _____ skills are essential in the psychiatric care setting.

4. _____ therapy involves sending an electric shock through the brain.

5. A person with _____ has trouble separating the real from the imaginary.

CHAPTER 14

Introduction to Medication Administration

SCOPE OF PRACTICE

Key Learning Point

- A nursing assistant's scope of practice in medication administration

Activity A *Place an "X" next to each correct answer for the following question.*

1. Which of the following health care personnel may write orders for medications?

    a. _____ Unlicensed assistive personnel

    b. _____ Nursing assistants

    c. _____ Physician assistants

    d. _____ Dentists

    e. _____ Nurse practitioners

Activity B *Think About It! Briefly answer the following question in the space provided.*

List three things a nursing assistant should verify before administering any medication.

_____

_____

_____

MEDICATION ADMINISTRATION ROUTES

Key Learning Point

- Different routes of medication administration

Activity C *Fill in the blanks using the words given in brackets.*

[topical, route, suppositories, sublingual, tablets]

1. The _____ is the way the person receives the medication.

2. Medications given by the oral route may take the form of liquids, _____, or capsules.

3. _____ medications are usually liquids or small, rapidly dissolving tablets that are absorbed through the mucous membrane of the mouth.

4. _____ medications are applied to the skin or mucous membranes.

5. _____ are placed in the rectum or vagina.

Activity D *Identify the devices shown in the figure. What are they used for?*

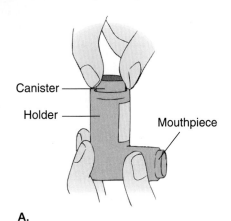

Canister
Holder
Mouthpiece

A.

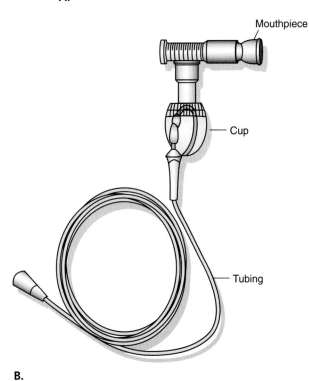

Mouthpiece
Cup
Tubing

B.

_____

_____

_____

Activity E *Match the type of injection, given in Column A with its administration method given in Column B.*

Column A

_____ **1.** Intradermal injection

_____ **2.** Subcutaneous injection

_____ **3.** Intramuscular injection

_____ **4.** Intravenous injection

Column B

a. Medications are injected into the fatty tissue.

b. Medications are placed directly into the bloodstream.

c. Medications are injected into the skin.

d. Medications are injected into the muscle.

SAFE MEDICATION ADMINISTRATION

Key Learning Points

■ Six rights of medication administration
■ Documentation of medication administration
■ The appropriate way to handle a medication error

Activity F *Think About It! Briefly answer the following question in the space provided.*

List five medication administration errors.

_____

_____

_____

Activity G *Place an "X" next to each correct answer for the following question.*

1. Which of the following are the rights of medication administration?

a. _____ Right time

b. _____ Right documentation

c. _____ Right diagnosis

d. _____ Right dose

e. _____ Right attention

Activity H *Think About It! Briefly answer the following question in the space provided.*

It is important to check the information on the medication label to make sure it matches the medication order. List the three times you should check the medication label to help avoid medication errors.

_____

_____

_____

Activity I *Fill in the blanks using the words given in brackets.*

[generic, brand, dose, chemical]

1. The _____ name describes the medication's molecular structure.

2. The _____ name is a medication's official name.

3. The _____ name is the name given to the medication by the manufacturer for marketing purposes.

4. The _____ is the amount of medication that the person is supposed to receive.

Activity J *Match the abbreviations given in Column A with their expanded forms given in Column B.*

Column A

____ 1. mcg
____ 2. mg
____ 3. gtts
____ 4. mEq
____ 5. mL

Column B

a. Milligram
b. Drops
c. Micrograms
d. Milliliter
e. Milliequivalent

Activity K *What is the medication administration record (MAR) used for?*

_____

_____

_____

Activity L *Match the abbreviations given in Column A with their appropriate descriptions given in Column B.*

Column A

____ 1. Ac
____ 2. BID
____ 3. TID
____ 4. PR
____ 5. PO

Column B

a. Oral administration
b. Before meals
c. Three times per day
d. Twice daily
e. Rectal administration

Activity M *Select the single best answer for the following question.*

1. A nursing assistant caring for a patient has administered a higher dose of medication to the patient than required. What step should the nursing assistant take immediately?

a. Inform the patient and apologize for the mistake.
b. Report the error to the nurse only if the patient starts to have problems.
c. Report to the nurse and document the error in an incident report.
d. Ignore it if the patient seems alright and be more careful the next time.

MEDICATION ADMINISTRATION SKILLS

Key Learning Points

- Different types of medication supply systems
- Proper way to prepare and administer an oral medication
- Proper way to administer a transdermal patch
- Proper way to administer eye drops
- Proper way to administer ear drops
- Proper way to insert a rectal suppository

Activity N *Fill in the blanks using the words given in brackets.*

[controlled, bubble pack, pill box, medicine bottle]

1. A _____ has compartments to store medication for each day of the week, each time of day, or both.

2. A _____ contains the patient's or resident's medication for a given amount of time.

3. A _____ is a flat card containing 15 to 30 doses of a medication for a single patient or resident.

4. _____ substances are often stored in computer-operated automated drawer systems and accounted for at the end of each shift.

Activity O *Think About It! Briefly answer the following question in the space provided.*

When administering medications, what observations should be reported to the nurse immediately?

_____

_____

_____

Activity P *Match the terms related to medication administration given in Column A with their appropriate descriptions given in Column B.*

Column A

_____ **1.** Medication cup

_____ **2.** Enteric coating

_____ **3.** Sustained-release preparations

_____ **4.** Pill splitter

_____ **5.** Medication-crushing device

Column B

a. Used to crush a tablet into a fine powder

b. Used to evenly split a tablet

c. Used for dispensing oral medications

d. A waxy layer on the outside of a tablet or capsule

e. Medication that is released slowly over an extended period

Activity Q *Match the medications given in Column A with their descriptions given in Column B.*

Column A

_____ **1.** Creams and ointments

_____ **2.** Transdermal patch

_____ **3.** Eye drops

_____ **4.** Suppository

_____ **5.** Enema

Column B

a. A small piece of adhesive material that contains a medication

b. Introduction of fluid into the large intestine by way of the anus

c. Used to treat rashes and other skin conditions

d. Used to treat eye conditions, such as glaucoma

e. Small, wax-like cone or oval that is inserted into the vagina or rectum

Activity R *Place an "X" next to each correct answer for the following questions.*

1. When administering an enema to a patient, which of the following should be done if the patient complains of dizziness and weakness?

   a. _____ Stop the enema

   b. _____ Place the person in supine position

   c. _____ Take vital signs

   d. _____ Give hot fluids to drink

   e. _____ Administer oxygen

Activity S *Write down the correct sequence of administering inhaled medications in the boxes provided below.*

1. Hold the mouthpiece of the inhaler 1 to 2 inches away from the mouth.

2. Press down on the canister to release the dose of medication.

3. Exhale through the mouth.

4. Take a deep breath and let out all the air.

5. Hold breath for about 10 seconds.

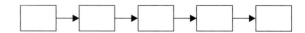

Activity T *Identify the device in the figure and state its use.*

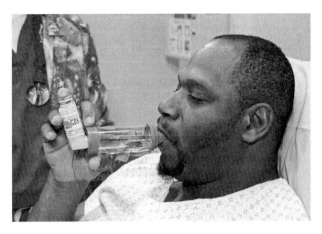

_____

_____

_____

Activity U *Select the single best answer for each of the following questions.*

1. The amount of fluid administered through an

   intradermal injection is _____.
   a. Less than 0.1 mL
   b. Up to 1 mL
   c. Up to 3 mL
   d. 5 mL

2. If medication that is intended for an intramuscular injection is administered into the subcutaneous tissue instead of the muscle, which of the following complications may occur?
   a. Vomiting
   b. Headache
   c. Tissue necrosis
   d. Chest pain

SUMMARY

Activity V *Match the medication administration routes given in Column A with their appropriate descriptions given in Column B.*

Column A

_____ 1. Oral route

_____ 2. Sublingual route

_____ 3. Topical route

_____ 4. Respiratory route

_____ 5. Parenteral route

Column B

a. Medications are injected into the body.

b. Medications are inhaled into the lungs.

c. Medications are swallowed.

d. Medications are placed under the tongue and allowed to dissolve.

e. Medications are applied to the skin or mucous membranes.

Activity W *Think About It! Briefly answer the following question in the space provided.*

List the six rights of medication administration that should be followed to prevent medication administration errors.

_____

_____

_____

15

Common Medications

MEDICATIONS USED TO RELIEVE PAIN

Key Learning Point

■ Two main types of pain medications and safety precautions related to their use

Activity A *Fill in the blanks using the words given in brackets.*

[analgesics, acute, side, chronic, therapeutic]

1. The intended effect of a medication is called its _____ effect.

2. The additional, unwanted effects of a medication on the body are called _____ effects.

3. _____ pain lasts for a short period of time and decreases as the body heals.

4. _____ pain is lasting pain.

5. Medications used to treat pain are often called _____.

Activity B *Select the single best answer for the following question.*

1. Narcotic analgesics work by _____.
   a. Increasing the blood circulation to the diseased body part
   b. Acting on opioid receptors in the brain, spinal cord, and gastrointestinal tract
   c. Temporarily controlling symptoms, such as vomiting
   d. Increasing the secretion of digestive juices in the stomach

Activity C *Identify the device shown in the figure below and state its use.*

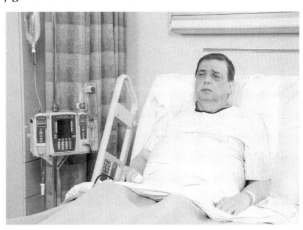

_____

_____

_____

Activity D *Place an "X" next to each correct answer for the following question.*

1. A nursing assistant is caring for a patient who is receiving narcotic analgesics for post-operative pain relief. Which of the following may be side effects of narcotic analgesics?
   a. _____ Increased respiratory rate
   b. _____ Anorexia
   c. _____ Drowsiness
   d. _____ Nausea
   e. _____ Diarrhea

Activity E *Think About It! Briefly answer the following question in the space provided.*

A nursing assistant is caring for a patient who is receiving a narcotic analgesic for pain relief. List the observations that the nursing assistant should report to the nurse immediately.

_____

_____

_____

Activity F *Select the single best answer for the following question.*

1. A nursing assistant trained in medication administration has to administer morphine to a patient. What should the nursing assistant do before administering the morphine?

   a. Measure the blood pressure.

   b. Measure the respiratory rate.

   c. Measure the temperature.

   d. Measure the weight.

2. Which of the following statements is true about non-narcotic analgesics?

   a. They are used to treat severe pain.

   b. They act through opioid receptors.

   c. They can also be used to lower fever.

   d. They frequently cause addiction in users.

Activity G *Fill in the blanks using the words given in brackets.*

[prostaglandins, stomach, reducing, bleeding]

1. NSAIDs relieve pain, inflammation, and fever

   by _____ the level of prostaglandins in the body.

2. _____ are hormone-like substances that act on different cells in the body to produce many different effects.

3. NSAIDs can irritate the lining of the

   _____, leading to ulcers and bleeding.

4. NSAIDs should not be used in people with

   _____ disorders because they affect the blood's ability to clot.

Activity H *Think About It! Briefly answer the following question in the space provided.*

You are caring for a patient who regularly takes aspirin for chronic arthritis pain. List the observations that you should immediately report to the nurse.

_____

_____

_____

Activity I *Select the single best answer for the following question.*

1. A nursing assistant is caring for a patient who has been prescribed acetaminophen as needed for pain. Acetaminophen is supplied to the patient in 500-mg tablets. Because too much acetaminophen can damage the liver, what is the maximum number of tablets the patient can have in a day?

   a. Two

   b. Four

   c. Six

   d. Eight

Activity J *Place an "N" next to the narcotic analgesics and an "NN" next to the non-narcotic analgesics.*

1. _____ Oxycodone

2. _____ Aspirin

3. _____ Ibuprofen

4. _____ Codeine

5. _____ Acetaminophen

6. _____ Fentanyl

MEDICATIONS USED TO SUPPRESS THE IMMUNE RESPONSE

Key Learning Points

■ The reasons why a person might be treated with corticosteroids

■ Side effects a nursing assistant should be observant for when caring for a person taking these medications

Activity K *Place an "X" next to each correct answer for the following question.*

1. For which of the following conditions are corticosteroid medications commonly used?

   a. _____ Addison's disease

   b. _____ Allergic reactions

   c. _____ Fracture

   d. _____ Fever

   e. _____ Rheumatoid arthritis

Activity L *Think About It! Briefly answer the following question in the space provided.*

A nursing assistant is caring for a patient undergoing treatment with corticosteroids. List some common side effects of this treatment.

_____

_____

_____

MEDICATIONS USED TO TREAT BACTERIAL INFECTIONS

Key Learning Points

- Reasons why a person might be treated with antibiotics
- Considerations that should be taken into account when caring for a person who is receiving antibiotics

Activity M *Select the single best answer for each of the following questions.*

1. Which of the following statements is true regarding antibiotic use?

   a. They are used to treat infections caused by bacteria.

   b. They are used only when the patient is allergic to other medications.

   c. They can be administered only through the intravenous route.

   d. Patient allergies are of no concern when administering antibiotics.

2. Which vital sign measurement is especially important for the nursing assistant to monitor closely when caring for a patient who is being treated with oral antibiotics?

   a. Blood pressure

   b. Respiration

   c. Temperature

   d. Oxygen saturation

Activity N *Think About It! Briefly answer the following question in the space provided.*

Why is it important to administer antibiotics at regular intervals?

_____

_____

_____

Activity O *Match the number of antibiotic doses ordered for each 24-hour period given in Column A with the appropriate hourly schedule given in Column B.*

Column A	Column B
_____ 1. One dose	a. Every 12 hours
_____ 2. Two doses	b. Every 6 hours
_____ 3. Three doses	c. Every 4 hours
_____ 4. Four doses	d. Every 24 hours
_____ 5. Six doses	e. Every 8 hours

Activity P *Think About It! Briefly answer the following questions in the space provided.*

1. Antibiotics may cause allergic reactions. What should the nursing assistant do before administering an antibiotic to a patient to help avoid an allergic reaction?

_____

_____

_____

2. List the signs and symptoms of allergic reactions to an antibiotic that should be reported to the nurse immediately.

_____

_____

_____

MEDICATIONS USED TO TREAT RESPIRATORY DISORDERS

Key Learning Points

- Reasons why a person might be treated with a bronchodilator
- Side effects for which a nursing assistant should be observant when caring for a person taking a bronchodilator

Activity Q *Write down the correct sequence of the action of bronchodilators in the boxes provided below.*

1. Administration of bronchodilators

2. Dilation of the airway

3. Relaxation of the smooth muscles of the bronchi and bronchioles

4. Easy movement of air through the airway

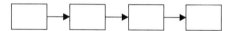

Activity R *Place an "L" next to the characteristics of long-acting bronchodilators and an "S" next to the characteristics of short-acting bronchodilators.*

1. _____ They are taken on a regular basis.

2. _____ They are often found in "rescue" inhalers.

3. _____ They are used on an as-needed basis.

4. _____ They often are a combination of a bronchodilator with a corticosteroid.

Activity S *Think About It! Briefly answer the following question in the space provided.*

A nursing assistant is caring for a patient undergoing treatment with bronchodilators for chronic obstructive pulmonary disorder. List the signs or symptoms that may indicate that the patient is developing side effects of bronchodilators.

_____

_____

_____

MEDICATIONS USED TO TREAT CARDIOVASCULAR DISORDERS

Key Learning Points

- Reasons why a person might be treated with an antihypertensive and safety precautions related to the use of antihypertensives
- Reasons why a person might be treated with nitroglycerin and safety precautions related to the use of nitroglycerin
- Reasons why a person might be treated with a cardiotonic and safety precautions related to the use of cardiotonics
- Reasons why a person might be treated with an anticoagulant and safety precautions related to the use of anticoagulants

Activity T *Place an "X" next to each correct answer for the following question.*

1. Which of the following statements are true about hypertension?

    a. _____ A low sodium diet has no effect on hypertension.

    b. _____ Systolic blood pressure is consistently higher than 140 mm Hg.

    c. _____ Diastolic blood pressure is consistently higher than 90 mm Hg.

    d. _____ A person with hypertension is at great risk for complications.

    e. _____ Physical exercises will not help hypertension.

Activity U *Think About It! Briefly answer the following questions in the space provided.*

1. List the blood pressure readings that should be reported to the nurse immediately when caring for a patient who is taking antihypertensive medications.

_____

_____

_____

2. A nursing assistant is caring for a patient who is receiving antihypertensive medications. List the observations, apart from blood pressure readings, that should be immediately reported to the nurse.

_____

_____

_____

Activity V *Think About It! Briefly answer the following question in the space provided.*

1. List the observations that the nursing assistant should immediately report to the nurse when caring for the patient receiving nitroglycerin.

_____

_____

_____

Activity W *Select the single best answer for the following question.*

1. A nursing assistant who has been trained in medication administration is administering nitroglycerin to a patient. Which of the following precautions should the nursing assistant take?

   a. Measure temperature before administering the medication.

   b. Wear gloves when handling the medication.

   c. Weigh the patient before administering the medication.

   d. Ask the patient if he is still having chest pain.

Activity X *Fill in the blanks using the words given in brackets.*

[digitalis, dysrhythmia, cardiotonics, slow]

1. Cardiotonics are medications that

   _____ the heart rate and increase the force of each heart beat.

2. _____ are frequently used in the treatment of atrial fibrillation.

3. Atrial fibrillation is a _____ that occurs when the atria sends too many impulses through the atrioventricular node, resulting in very fast and very irregular contraction of the ventricles.

4. Digoxin is made from the _____ plant.

Activity Y *What does the figure depict? Why is this procedure important for a patient receiving digoxin?*

_____

_____

_____

Activity Z *Place an "X" next to each correct answer for the following question.*

1. A nursing assistant is caring for a patient who has heart failure and is being treated with digoxin. Which of the following may be signs of digoxin toxicity?

   a. _____ Nausea or vomiting

   b. _____ Apical pulse rate is less than 60 beats/min

   c. _____ Unusual weight gain

   d. _____ Visual disturbances

   e. _____ Drowsiness

Activity AA *Fill in the blanks using the words given in brackets.*

[heparin, aspirin, warfarin, thrombus, anticoagulants]

1. _____ are medications that are given to prevent the blood from clotting.

2. _____ is an anticoagulant that is administered orally.

3. _____ is an anticoagulant that is administered parenterally.

4. Daily low doses of _____, a common analgesic, help prevent clot formation.

5. Surgery, stroke, and atrial fibrillation put a person at risk for _____ formation.

Activity AB *Think About It! Briefly answer the following questions in the space provided.*

1. What factors should the nursing assistant be aware of when caring for a patient who is prescribed the anticoagulant warfarin?

_____

_____

_____

2. When caring for a person who is taking an anticoagulant, what signs and symptoms should be reported immediately to the nurse?

_____

_____

_____

MEDICATIONS USED TO TREAT URINARY DISORDERS

Key Learning Points

- Reasons why a person might be treated with a diuretic and safety precautions related to the use of diuretics
- Reasons why a person might be treated with an antispasmodic and safety precautions related to the use of antispasmodics

Activity AC *Place an "X" next to each correct answer for the following questions.*

1. Which of the following conditions may be indications for diuretic use?
   a. ____ Surgery
   b. ____ Atrial fibrillation
   c. ____ Kidney disease
   d. ____ Congestive heart failure
   e. ____ Hypertension

2. A nursing assistant is caring for a patient who is taking furosemide and an oral potassium supplement. Which of the following conditions may suggest that the potassium level is low in the patient?
   a. ____ The pulse is irregular.
   b. ____ The patient complains of muscle weakness or muscle cramps.
   c. ____ The patient is dehydrated.
   d. ____ The patient has put on weight.
   e. ____ The patient complains of nausea and vomiting.

Activity AD *Think About It! Briefly answer the following questions in the space provided.*

1. What are the responsibilities of a nursing assistant when caring for a patient who is receiving diuretics?

_____

_____

_____

2. List the signs and symptoms that indicate that the diuretic may not be working properly.

_____

_____

_____

Activity AE *Fill in the blanks using the words given in brackets.*

[urge, cystitis, antispasmodics, involuntary]

1. Bladder spasms are _____ contractions of the smooth muscle in the walls of the bladder.

2. When the muscular walls of the bladder suddenly contract, urine is expelled from the body with little warning, resulting in _____ incontinence.

3. _____ is an infection of the bladder that can cause bladder spasms.

4. _____ are medications used to suppress contractions of the smooth muscle in the walls of hollow muscular organs.

MEDICATIONS USED TO TREAT GASTROINTESTINAL DISORDERS

Key Learning Point

■ Safety considerations related to the administration of medications used to treat diarrhea and constipation

Activity AF *Think About It! Briefly answer the following question in the space provided.*

What observations and precautions must the nursing assistant be aware of when caring for a patient who is prescribed Lomotil for loose stools?

_____

_____

_____

Activity AG *Following are examples of medications used to treat constipation. Place an "L" next to stimulant laxatives, an "S" next to stool softeners, and an "F" next to fiber supplements.*

1. _____ Psyllium

2. _____ Magnesium hydroxide

3. _____ Docusate calcium

4. _____ Polycarbophil

5. _____ Docusate sodium

6. _____ Senna

Activity AH *Fill in the blanks using the words given in brackets.*

[exercise, enema, diarrhea, orally]

1. Milk of Magnesia, a medication used to treat constipation, is administered _____.

2. When caring for a person who is taking a laxative, a stool softener, or a fiber supplement, encouraging fluid intake and _____ can help these medications work better.

3. A rectal suppository or a/an _____ may be ordered if medications do not relieve constipation.

4. Laxatives or fiber supplements are avoided if the patient is experiencing _____ or abdominal pain.

MEDICATIONS USED TO TREAT ENDOCRINE DISORDERS

Key Learning Points

■ Observations a nursing assistant may make that should be reported to the nurse when caring for a patient who is being treated with medication for hypothyroidism
■ Observations a nursing assistant may make that should be reported to the nurse when caring for a patient who is being treated with medication for diabetes

Activity AI *Select the single best answer for the following question.*

1. Hypothyroidism is caused by a deficiency of the hormone _____.
   a. Thyroxine
   b. Adrenaline
   c. Insulin
   d. Prolactin

Activity AJ *Place an "X" next to each correct answer for the following question.*

1. Which of the following are signs and symptoms of hypothyroidism?
   a. _____ Fatigue
   b. _____ Depression
   c. _____ Weight loss
   d. _____ Intolerance to heat
   e. _____ Constipation

Activity AK *Think About It! Briefly answer the following question in the space provided.*

A nursing assistant is caring for a patient who is taking medication for hypothyroidism. List the observations that the nursing assistant should report to the nurse.

_____

_____

_____

Activity AL *Match the terms related to diabetes mellitus given in Column A with their descriptions given in Column B.*

Column A

_____ 1. Type 1 diabetes mellitus

_____ 2. Type 2 diabetes mellitus

_____ 3. Short-acting insulins

_____ 4. Intermediate-acting insulins

_____ 5. Long-acting insulins

Column B

a. They start working within 1 to 2 hours, peak within 6 to 12 hours, and last 16 to 24 hours.

b. The insulin-producing cells of the pancreas are completely destroyed, and no insulin is produced.

c. They start working within 4 to 6 hours, peak within 10 to 18 hours, and last 24 or more hours.

d. They start working within 30 to 60 minutes, peak within 1 to 4 hours, and last 5 to 8 hours.

e. The insulin-producing cells of the pancreas still produce some insulin, but the cells of the body are not able to respond to the insulin.

Activity AM *Think About It! Briefly answer the following questions in the space provided.*

1. List signs and symptoms of hypoglycemia.

_____

_____

_____

2. What are the responsibilities of the nursing assistant when administering oral medications for diabetes?

_____

_____

_____

MEDICATIONS USED TO TREAT PSYCHIATRIC DISORDERS

Key Learning Point

■ Medications used to treat psychiatric disorders

Activity AN *Select the single best answer for the following question.*

1. Which of the following disorders is treated with anxiolytics?
   a. Depression
   b. Dementia
   c. Anxiety
   d. Schizophrenia

SUMMARY

Activity AO *Match the class of drugs given in Column A with their actions given in Column B.*

Column A

_____ 1. Analgesics

_____ 2. Corticosteroids

_____ 3. Antibiotics

_____ 4. Bronchodilators

_____ 5. Diuretics

_____ 6. Antihypertensives

_____ 7. Cardiotonics

_____ 8. Anticoagulants

_____ 9. Antispasmodics

Column B

a. Treats bacterial infections

b. Treats pain

c. Opens the airway

d. Increases the urine output

e. Suppresses the immune system

f. Prevents blood clots from forming in the cardiovascular system

g. Stops bladder spasms

h. Lowers the blood pressure

i. Slows the heart rate and increases the force of each heart beat, increasing cardiac output

Activity AP *Fill in the blanks using the words given in brackets.*

[Levothroid, Tylenol, nitroglycerin, Lomotil, digoxin, metformin]

1. _____ is used to treat diarrhea.

2. _____ is used to increase the flow of blood to the heart and relieve chest pain.

3. Hypothyroidism is treated with the daily administration of _____.

4. _____ is used to treat diabetes.

5. _____ should not be administered if the heart rate is less than 60 bpm.

6. _____ is an example of a non-narcotic analgesic.

CHAPTER 2 PROCEDURE CHECKLISTS

PROCEDURE 2-1

Creating a Sterile Field from an Envelope-Wrapped Package

	S	U	COMMENTS
1. Gather needed supplies: envelope-wrapped package that will form a sterile drape, disinfectant, paper towels.	☐	☐	_____
2. Use the disinfectant and paper towels to disinfect the work surface (for example, the over-bed table) and dry it thoroughly. Position the over-bed table at a comfortable working height.	☐	☐	_____
3. Wash your hands.	☐	☐	_____
4. Explain the procedure to the patient. Explain the importance of avoiding contamination of the sterile field. Ask the patient to avoid touching the sterile field.	☐	☐	_____
5. Verify that the item inside the envelope-style package is sterile by checking the outside of the package.			
a. If the package was processed on-site, check the chemical indicator on the outside of the package to make sure that it has changed.	☐	☐	_____
b. If the package was processed by the manufacturer, look for the statement on the outside of the package that indicates that the contents are sterile.	☐	☐	_____
c. Check the package for tears, holes, worn areas, and water spot discolorations. These findings indicate that the item inside the package is no longer sterile.	☐	☐	_____
6. If there is any indication that the items inside the package are not sterile, discard the package and obtain a new one. Otherwise, continue with the procedure.	☐	☐	_____
7. Place the package on the surface of your work area, in the center. Make sure the package is positioned so that the first flap will open away from you.	☐	☐	_____
8. Touching only the outer corner of the first flap, open the package away from you by reaching around (not over) it. Pull the flap firmly, straightening out the material so that the flap does not fold back onto the package. (If the flap folds back onto the package, the place where your fingers touched the flap will come in contact with the item inside the package, contaminating it.)	☐	☐	_____
9. Touching only the outer corner of the left flap, open it to the left. Pull the flap firmly, straightening out the material so that the flap does not fold back onto the package.	☐	☐	_____

10. Touching only the outer corner of the right flap, open it to the right. Pull the flap firmly, straightening out the material so that the flap does not fold back onto the package.   ☐ ☐ _____

11. Touching only the outer corner of the last flap, open it toward you. Pull the flap firmly, straightening out the material so that the flap does not fold back onto the package.   ☐ ☐ _____

PROCEDURE 2-2
Creating a Sterile Field Using a Sterile Drape

	S	U	COMMENTS

1. Gather needed supplies: package containing sterile drape, disinfectant, paper towels   ☐ ☐ _____

2. Use the disinfectant and paper towels to disinfect the work surface (for example, the over-bed table) and dry it thoroughly. Position the over-bed table at a comfortable working height.   ☐ ☐ _____

3. Wash your hands.   ☐ ☐ _____

4. Explain the procedure to the patient. Explain the importance of avoiding contamination of the sterile field. Ask the patient to avoid touching the sterile field.   ☐ ☐ _____

5. Verify that the sterile drape inside the package is sterile by checking the outside of the package.

   a. If the package was processed on-site, check the chemical indicator on the outside of the package to make sure that it has changed.   ☐ ☐ _____

   b. If the package was processed by the manufacturer, look for the statement on the outside of the package that indicates that the contents are sterile.   ☐ ☐ _____

   c. Check the package for tears, holes, worn areas, and water spot discolorations. These findings indicate that the item inside the package is no longer sterile.   ☐ ☐ _____

6. If there is any indication that the sterile drape inside the package is not sterile, discard the package and obtain a new one. Otherwise, continue with the procedure.   ☐ ☐ _____

7. Open the package containing the drape.

   a. If the package is wrapped envelope style, place the package flat on the clean work surface and open it in the manner described in Procedure 2-1.   ☐ ☐ _____

   b. If the package is a peel pouch, place the package flat on the clean work surface. Peel the top flap back while holding the bottom flap steady until the package is flat against the work surface. Make sure to open the package fully so that the top flap of the package does not fold back down over the sterile drape. (If the top flap folds back down over the sterile drape, the place where your fingers touched the package will come in contact with the drape inside the package, contaminating it.)   ☐ ☐ _____

8. Look for the edge of the sterile drape that is folded back to create a small area for you to grasp.   ☐ ☐ _____

9. Grasp the edge of the drape with your thumb and index finger and lift the sterile drape straight up as you step back. Do not allow the sterile drape to drag across the wrapper as you lift it up.

☐ ☐ _____

10. Hold the sterile drape away from your body and allow it to unfold. Do not shake the sterile drape. Grasp the other top corner of the sterile drape with the thumb and index finger of your other hand and allow the sterile drape to unfold completely. Make sure that the drape does not touch your arms, your uniform, or other surfaces and make sure to only hold the sterile drape at the edges.

☐ ☐ _____

11. When the sterile drape is unfolded completely, turn carefully toward the work surface that you plan to drape. Holding the sterile drape up high, place the sterile drape across the work surface, starting with the edge of the work surface that is farthest away from you. This way, you do not reach across the sterile field or risk moving the front of your body too close to it.

☐ ☐ _____

PROCEDURE 2-3
Adding Envelope-Wrapped Sterile Items to the Sterile Field

	S	U	COMMENTS

1. Gather needed supplies: envelope-wrapped package that will form a sterile drape OR package containing a sterile drape (to create the sterile field), envelope-wrapped package containing sterile item to be added to the sterile field.   ☐ ☐ _____

2. Create a sterile field (see Procedures 2-1 and 2-2).   ☐ ☐ _____

3. Verify that the item inside the package is sterile by checking the outside of the package.

   a. If the package was processed on-site, check the chemical indicator on the outside of the package to make sure that it has changed.   ☐ ☐ _____

   b. If the package was processed by the manufacturer, look for the statement on the outside of the package that indicates that the contents are sterile.   ☐ ☐ _____

   c. Check the package for tears, holes, worn areas, and water spot discolorations. These findings indicate that the item inside the package is no longer sterile.   ☐ ☐ _____

4. If there is any indication that the item inside the package is not sterile, discard the package and obtain a new one. Otherwise, continue with the procedure.   ☐ ☐ _____

5. Stand back from the sterile field and hold the bottom edge of the package in one hand. Make sure the package is positioned so that the first flap will open away from you.   ☐ ☐ _____

6. Touching only the outer corner of the first flap with your other hand, open it away from you by reaching around (not over) the package. Pull the flap firmly, straightening out the material so that the flap does not fold back onto the package. (If the flap folds back onto the package, the place where your fingers touched the flap will come in contact with the item inside the package, contaminating it.)   ☐ ☐ _____

7. Touching only the outer corner of the left flap, open it to the left. Pull the flap firmly, straightening out the material so that the flap does not fold back onto the package.   ☐ ☐ _____

8. Touching only the outer corner of the right flap, open it to the right. Pull the flap firmly, straightening out the material so that the flap does not fold back onto the package.   ☐ ☐ _____

9. Touching only the outer corner of the last flap, open it toward you, covering the hand holding the item. Pull the flap firmly, straightening out the material so that the flap does not fold back onto the package.   ☐ ☐ _____

10. Holding the item securely, gather the corners of all four flaps around your wrist with your other hand so that your hand and wrist are covered. Avoid touching the inside of the wrapper. ☐ ☐ _____

11. Step toward the sterile field. Extend your hands, holding the item about 6 inches above the sterile field. Turn your hands over and gently drop the item out of the wrapper onto the center of the sterile field. (Remember that the outer 1 inch of the field is considered contaminated.) ☐ ☐ _____

12. Dispose of the wrapper in a facility-approved waste container. ☐ ☐ _____

PROCEDURE 2-4
Adding Sterile Items That Are Contained in a Peel Pouch to a Sterile Field

	S	U	COMMENTS

1. Gather needed supplies: envelope-wrapped package that will form a sterile drape or package containing a sterile drape (to create the sterile field), sterile item contained in a peel pouch to be added to the sterile field ☐ ☐ _____

2. Create a sterile field (see Procedures 2-1 and 2-2). ☐ ☐ _____

3. Verify that the item inside the package is sterile by checking the outside of the package.

   a. If the package was processed on-site, check the chemical indicator on the outside of the package to make sure that it has changed. ☐ ☐ _____

   b. If the package was processed by the manufacturer, look for the statement on the outside of the package that indicates that the contents are sterile. ☐ ☐ _____

   c. Check the package for tears, holes, worn areas, and water spot discolorations. These findings indicate that the item inside the package is no longer sterile. ☐ ☐ _____

4. If there is any indication that the item inside the package is not sterile, discard the package and obtain a new one. Otherwise, continue with the procedure. ☐ ☐ _____

5. Stand back from the sterile field. Grasp the separate edges of the peel pouch between your thumbs and the gently folded fists of each hand. ☐ ☐ _____

6. Start pulling the edges of the peel pouch away from each other, separating the pouch along the edges. If the peel pouch tears down the center instead of separating along the edges, the item is considered contaminated, and you must discard it. ☐ ☐ _____

7. As you open the peel pouch, hold it so that one side becomes the bottom and the other becomes the top. The sterile item will be lying on the bottom flap until the package is opened completely. ☐ ☐ _____

8. Step toward the sterile field. Hold the peel pouch over the sterile field at about a height of 6 inches. Flip the item onto the center of the sterile field by bringing the hand that is holding the bottom flap down and back while you bring the hand that is holding the upper flap up and over. (Remember that the outer 1 inch of the field is considered contaminated.) Do not allow the item to touch the edges of the peel pouch, which are also considered contaminated. ☐ ☐ _____

9. Dispose of the peel pouch in a facility-approved waste container. ☐ ☐ _____

PROCEDURE 2-5
Pouring a Sterile Solution into a Sterile Container

	S	U	COMMENTS

1. Gather needed supplies: envelope-wrapped package that will form a sterile drape or package containing a sterile drape (to create the sterile field), envelope-wrapped package containing small sterile basin or peel-pack package containing a sterile cup (such as a sterile specimen cup), bottle of sterile solution ☐ ☐ _____

2. Create a sterile field (see Procedures 2-1 and 2-2). ☐ ☐ _____

3. Add the sterile basin or cup to the sterile field (see Procedures 2-3 and 2-4). If necessary, use transfer forceps or sterile gloves to position the sterile basin or cup right side up, close to the outside edge of the sterile field. (Remember that the outer 1 inch of the field is considered contaminated.) ☐ ☐ _____

4. Carefully check the label on the bottle of sterile solution. Make sure it is the correct solution and the correct strength. Also note the expiration date or "use by" date.

   a. **Multiple-use bottles.** Antibacterial solutions (such as Betadine, alcohol, hydrogen peroxide, or prepping solution) are often supplied in multiple-use bottles. Multiple-use bottles should be labeled with the time and date they were opened for the first time. ☐ ☐ _____

   b. **Single-use bottles.** Normal saline and sterile water are usually supplied in single-use bottles. Single-use bottles should not be recapped for use later. Follow your facility policy. ☐ ☐ _____

5. Check the bottle for cracks, a broken lid seal, and discoloration of the solution. If there is any indication that the sterile solution is not sterile, discard the bottle and obtain a new one. Otherwise, continue with the procedure. ☐ ☐ _____

6. Open the bottle of sterile solution. Place the cap on a clean surface with the inside of the cap facing up. Be careful not to touch the inside of the cap. ☐ ☐ _____

7. If the solution is contained in a multiple-use bottle that has been opened previously, pour a small amount of the solution into the waste container to cleanse the lip of the bottle. This procedure is known as "lipping." ☐ ☐ _____

8. Without reaching over the sterile field, hold the tip of the bottle about 4 to 6 inches above the sterile basin or cup and carefully pour the required amount of solution into it. Avoid splashing liquid onto the sterile drape. ☐ ☐ _____

9. If solution remains in a multiple-use bottle, recap the bottle, being careful to touch only the outside of the cap. Dispose of a single-use bottle or an empty multiple-use bottle in a facility-approved waste container.

☐ ☐ _____

PROCEDURE 2-6
Putting On and Removing Sterile Gloves

Putting On Sterile Gloves

	S	U	COMMENTS
1. Gather needed supplies: sterile gloves in the appropriate size	☐	☐	_____
2. Wash your hands.	☐	☐	_____
3. Verify that the gloves inside the package are sterile by checking the outside of the package.			
a. Look for the statement on the outside of the package that indicates that the contents are sterile.	☐	☐	_____
b. Check the package for tears, holes, worn areas, and water spot discolorations. These findings indicate that the gloves inside the package are no longer sterile.	☐	☐	_____
4. If there is any indication that the gloves inside the package are not sterile, discard the package and obtain a new one. Otherwise, continue with the procedure.	☐	☐	_____
5. Open the outer wrapper by peeling it apart to expose the inner package. Remove the inner package, touching only the outside of it.	☐	☐	_____
6. Dispose of the outer wrapper in a facility-approved waste container. Place the inner package on a clean, dry surface.	☐	☐	_____
7. Open the inner package by carefully grasping the center flaps and pulling them open to the sides. Do not touch the inside of the package. Pull the flaps firmly, straightening out the material so that the flaps do not fold back onto the gloves. If the flaps fold back onto the gloves, the places where your fingers touched the flaps will come in contact with the gloves, contaminating them.	☐	☐	_____
8. Fold the lower flap underneath the inner package. This helps hold the package open for you. Note that the gloves are positioned with the fingers pointing away from you and the cuffs toward you. The gloves are labeled *R* and *L* for the right and left hands, respectively.	☐	☐	_____
9. Using the thumb and index finger of your nondominant hand, grasp the folded edge of the cuff on the glove for the dominant hand. Do not touch the inside of the package.	☐	☐	_____
10. Lift the glove straight up. (Do not slide it across the package.) Take one step backward. Avoid letting the glove touch anything.	☐	☐	_____

11. Holding your hands above waist level, carefully insert your dominant hand, palm up, into the glove and slowly pull the glove on. Leave the cuff folded down. (Your bare fingers only come into contact with the part of the sterile glove that will contact bare skin.)　☐ ☐ _____

12. With your gloved hand, reach toward the remaining glove. Holding your thumb up and out of the way, slide your gloved fingers under the cuff of the remaining glove.　☐ ☐ _____

13. Lift the glove straight up. (Do not slide it across the package.) Take one step backward. Avoid letting the glove touch anything.　☐ ☐ _____

14. Holding your hands above waist level, carefully insert your nondominant hand, palm up, into the glove and slowly pull on the glove. Do not allow the thumb of your dominant hand to touch the skin of your nondominant hand as you are putting on the glove.　☐ ☐ _____

15. Keeping your fingers underneath the cuff, pull the cuff up over your wrist. Be careful not to touch the skin on your arm with your gloved hand.　☐ ☐ _____

16. Insert the gloved fingers of your nondominant hand under the cuff of the glove on your dominant hand (which is still folded). Pull the cuff up over your wrist. (Your gloved fingers only come into contact with the part of the sterile glove that did not contact bare skin.)　☐ ☐ _____

17. Adjust the gloves on both hands, touching only sterile areas. Pull the fingers of the gloves down so that excess glove material is not wrinkled over your fingertips.　☐ ☐ _____

Removing Sterile Gloves

1. With one gloved hand, grasp the other glove at the palm and pull the glove off your hand. Keep the glove you have removed in your gloved hand. (Think "glove to glove.")　☐ ☐ _____

2. Slip two fingers from the ungloved hand underneath the cuff of the remaining glove at the wrist. Remove that glove from your hand, turning it inside out as you pull it off. (Think "skin to skin.")　☐ ☐ _____

3. Dispose of the soiled gloves in a facility-approved waste container.　☐ ☐ _____

4. Wash your hands.　☐ ☐ _____

CHAPTER 3 PROCEDURE CHECKLISTS

PROCEDURE 3-1
Cleaning a Wound and Applying a Sterile Dressing

	S	U	COMMENTS

Getting Ready

1. Complete the "Getting Ready" steps. ☐ ☐ _____

Procedure

2. Place the dressing supplies on a clean surface, such as the bedside table. ☐ ☐ _____

3. Make sure that the bed is positioned at a comfortable working height (to promote good body mechanics) and that the wheels are locked. ☐ ☐ _____

4. If the side rails are in use, lower the side rail on the working side of the bed. The side rail on the opposite side of the bed should remain up. ☐ ☐ _____

5. Help the person to a comfortable position that allows access to the wound. ☐ ☐ _____

6. Fanfold the top linens to the foot of the bed. Adjust the person's hospital gown or pajamas as necessary to expose the wound. If necessary, use a bath blanket to provide additional warmth and modesty, leaving only the wound exposed. If necessary, place the bed protector under the wound site to keep the linens dry. ☐ ☐ _____

7. Fold down the top edges of the plastic bag to make a cuff. Place the cuffed bag on the over-bed table. ☐ ☐ _____

8. Put on the non-sterile gloves. ☐ ☐ _____

9. Loosen the tape that is securing the old dressing to the skin and remove the tape gently. Using a peeling action, carefully remove the soiled dressing. If the dressing sticks to the wound, apply a small amount of sterile saline to the dressing to moisten it. This will make the dressing easier to remove. ☐ ☐ _____

10. Being careful to keep the soiled side of the dressing out of the person's sight, observe the dressing for the amount, color, and odor of any drainage. Place the soiled dressing in the cuffed plastic bag. Do not let the dressing touch the outside of the bag. ☐ ☐ _____

11. Remove your gloves and dispose of them in a facility-approved waste container. ☐ ☐ _____

12. If the side rails are in use, return them to the raised position. ☐ ☐ _____

13. Wash your hands. ☐ ☐ _____

14. If the side rails are in use, lower the side rail on the working side of the bed. ☐ ☐ _____

15. Create the sterile field on the over-bed table using the sterile drape. ☐ ☐ _____

16. Add the sterile items to the sterile field:

   a. Open the sterile dressing set onto the sterile field. ☐ ☐ _____

   b. Open the sterile dressings onto the sterile field. ☐ ☐ _____

   c. Open the sterile gauze sponges onto the sterile field. ☐ ☐ _____

   d. Open the sterile basin onto the sterile field. ☐ ☐ _____

   e. Open the sterile saline and pour some into the sterile basin. ☐ ☐ _____

   f. If needed, open the sterile bulb syringe onto the sterile field. ☐ ☐ _____

17. Put on the sterile gloves. ☐ ☐ _____

18. Clean the wound.

   a. **If there is no drain:** Pick up a gauze sponge using your gloved hands or sponge forceps. Moisten the gauze sponge with the sterile saline by dipping it into the basin. Place the saline-soaked gauze sponge at the top of the incision site and stroke downward. Place the soiled gauze sponge in the cuffed plastic bag, being careful not to touch the bag. Clean each side of the wound in the same manner using a clean saline-soaked gauze sponge for each stroke. ☐ ☐ _____

   b. **If there is a drain:** Pick up a gauze sponge using your gloved hands or sponge forceps. Moisten the gauze sponge with the sterile saline by dipping it into the basin. Place the saline-soaked gauze sponge next to the drain and move it in a circular motion around the drain. Move outward from the drain using a clean saline-soaked gauze sponge for each stroke. ☐ ☐ _____

   c. **If the wound is to be irrigated (rinsed):** Hold several gauze sponges on the skin near the wound (to absorb the saline as it flows out of the wound). Draw up saline in the sterile bulb syringe and gently irrigate the wound. When you have finished irrigating the wound, place the sterile bulb syringe back in the basin and place the soiled gauze sponges in the cuffed plastic bag, being careful not to touch the bag. ☐ ☐ _____

19. Dry the wound using dry gauze sponges. Stroke from top to bottom or in a circular motion in the same manner that you used to clean the wound, using a clean gauze sponge for each stroke. ☐ ☐ _____

20. Observe the wound and surrounding tissues. Call the nurse to the bedside if you notice anything that may indicate an infection or separation of the wound edges. ☐ ☐ _____

21. If a medication or ointment has been ordered, apply it to the wound edges. ☐ ☐ _____

22. Apply the contact layer of the sterile dressing to the wound. If a drain is in place, use sterile scissors to cut a slit in the contact layer so it will fit around the drain site before placing the contact layer on the wound. ☐ ☐ _____

23. Apply the secondary layer of the sterile dressing to the wound. ☐ ☐ _____

24. Remove the sterile gloves. Put on a clean pair of non-sterile gloves. ☐ ☐ _____

25. If the dressing will be secured with tape, cut four pieces of tape for securing the dressing. The tape should be long enough to extend 2 inches past the dressing material on each side. Hang the tape from the edge of the over-bed table. ☐ ☐ _____

26. Use the tape strips to secure the dressing by placing one piece of tape along each side of the dressing. Center each piece of tape equally over the dressing and the person's skin. ☐ ☐ _____

27. Remove your gloves and dispose of them in a facility-approved waste container. Wash your hands. ☐ ☐ _____

28. Re-cover the wounded area with the person's hospital gown or pajamas. Help him back into a comfortable position, straighten the bottom linens, and draw the top linens over the person. ☐ ☐ _____

29. Make sure that the bed is lowered to its lowest position and that the wheels are locked. If the side rails are in use, return them to the raised position on the working side of the bed. ☐ ☐ _____

30. Dispose of disposable items in a facility-approved waste container. Clean the equipment and return it to the area designated by your facility. ☐ ☐ _____

Finishing Up

31. Complete the "Finishing Up" steps. ☐ ☐ _____

CHAPTER 4 PROCEDURE CHECKLISTS

PROCEDURE 4-1
Inserting a Straight Urinary Catheter

	S	U	COMMENTS

Getting Ready

1. Complete the "Getting Ready" steps. ☐ ☐ _____

Procedure

2. Place the catheterization supplies on a clean surface, such as the bedside table. ☐ ☐ _____

3. Make sure that the bed is positioned at a comfortable working height (to promote good body mechanics) and that the wheels are locked. Lower the head of the bed to a flat position (as tolerated). If the side rails are in use, lower the rail on the working side of the bed. The side rail on the opposite side of the bed should remain up. ☐ ☐ _____

4. Fanfold the linens to the foot of the bed. Position the person on his or her back. If the person is a woman, have her spread her legs apart and bend her knees slightly, if possible. (A woman can also be positioned on her side with her knees drawn to her chest.) Adjust the person's hospital gown or pajamas as necessary to expose the perineal area. Drape the person with the bath blanket. Position the bed protector under the person's buttocks to keep the bed linens dry. ☐ ☐ _____

5. Put on the non-sterile gloves and provide perineal care. ☐ ☐ _____

6. Dispose of the bed protector in a facility-approved waste container. Cover the perineal area, remove your gloves and dispose of them in a facility-approved waste container, and wash your hands. (If the side rails are in use, raise them before leaving the bedside.) ☐ ☐ _____

7. Return to the bedside. If the side rails are in use, lower the side rail on the working side of the bed. Expose the person's perineal area before creating your sterile field. ☐ ☐ _____

8. Using sterile technique, create a sterile field by opening the urinary catheter insertion kit on the work surface. (The paper wrapper becomes the sterile field.) ☐ ☐ _____

9. Remove the sterile glove package without touching the other items inside the urinary catheter insertion kit. Place the sterile glove package on the work surface next to the urinary catheter insertion kit. ☐ ☐ _____

10. **Position the first drape (the one without the opening).** Look for the edge of the sterile drape that is folded back to create a small area for you to grasp. Grasp the edge of the sterile drape with your thumb and index finger and lift the sterile drape straight up as you step back. Hold the sterile drape away from your body and allow it to unfold. Grasp the other top corner of the sterile drape with the thumb and index finger of your other hand and allow the sterile drape to unfold completely.

   a. Carefully fold the sterile drape in half lengthwise so that the sterile side is covering itself. ☐ ☐ _____

   b. Open the drape. The non-sterile side will be resting on your forearms. ☐ ☐ _____

   c. Ask the person to lift the buttocks. Position the sterile drape on the bed just under the buttocks with the sterile side facing up. Pull your arms out from under the sterile drape, being careful not to lean or reach over the sterile drape. ☐ ☐ _____

11. Put on the sterile gloves. ☐ ☐ _____

12. If needed, set up the specimen container by loosening or removing the lid. Leave the specimen container and lid on the sterile field. ☐ ☐ _____

13. **Position the fenestrated drape (if used).** Look for the edge of the sterile drape that is folded back to create a small area for you to grasp. Grasp the edge of the sterile drape with your thumb and index finger and lift the sterile drape straight up as you step back. Hold the sterile drape away from your body and allow it to unfold. Grasp the other top corner of the sterile drape with the thumb and index finger of your other hand and allow the sterile drape to unfold completely.

   a. **Female patient:** Position the sterile drape over the perineum so that the labia are exposed, being careful not to touch anything but the fenestrated drape with your sterile gloves. ☐ ☐ _____

   b. **Male patient:** Position the sterile drape with the opening over the penis, being careful not to touch anything but the fenestrated drape with your sterile gloves. ☐ ☐ _____

14. Pour antiseptic cleanser over the cotton balls or open the antiseptic cleansing swabs. ☐ ☐ _____

15. Open the packet of lubricant or uncap the lubricant syringe. Lubricate the tip of the catheter.

   a. **Female patient:** Lubricate 1 to 2 inches. ☐ ☐ _____

   b. **Male patient:** Lubricate 4 to 5 inches. ☐ ☐ _____

16. Clean the urinary meatus.   ☐ ☐ _____

   a. **Female patient:** Spread the labia apart using your non-dominant hand. (Your non-dominant hand is now contaminated.) Using your dominant hand, pick up an antiseptic swab or use the forceps to pick up an antiseptic-soaked cotton ball. Using a clean cotton ball or swab for each stroke, first clean one side, then the other side, and finally the middle, starting at the top and stroking downward. To avoid contaminating the meatus, you must continue to hold the labia apart until the catheter insertion is finished.

   b. **Male patient:** Hold the penis using your non-dominant hand. (Your non-dominant hand is now contaminated.) Using your dominant hand, pick up an antiseptic swab or use the forceps to pick up an antiseptic-soaked cotton ball.   ☐ ☐ _____

      • **If the man is circumcised:** Place the cotton ball or the antiseptic swab at the tip of the penis and stroke in a circular motion downward to the base of the penis. Repeat two more times using a clean cotton ball or swab for each stroke.

      • **If the man is uncircumcised:** Retract the foreskin by gently pushing the skin toward the base of the penis. Place the cotton ball or the antiseptic swab at the tip of the penis and stroke in a circular motion downward to the base of the penis. Repeat two more times using a clean cotton ball or swab for each stroke. To avoid contaminating the meatus, you must continue to retract the foreskin until the catheter insertion is finished.

17. Using your dominant hand, place the box holding the catheter between the person's legs. (The box will function as the basin to collect the urine.) Avoid touching the bed, the linens, or the person with your sterile dominant hand.   ☐ ☐ _____

18. Insert the urinary catheter. Pick up the catheter, holding it about 2 inches from the end. Leave the other end in the box.

   a. **Female patient:** Ask the patient to breathe deeply. Insert the catheter into the urinary meatus and advance it slowly until the catheter passes into the bladder and urine begins to flow (about 2 to 3 inches).   ☐ ☐ _____

      TIP: *If you are catheterizing a woman and urine does not begin to flow, you probably inserted the catheter into the vaginal opening instead of the urinary meatus. (It is easy to confuse the vaginal opening and the urinary meatus, especially in older women.) Leave the catheter in place, obtain new supplies, and begin again. Leaving the first catheter in place will make it easier to identify the urinary meatus on your second attempt.*

b. **Male patient:** Ask the patient to breathe deeply. Insert the catheter into the urinary meatus and advance it slowly until the catheter passes into the bladder and urine begins to flow (about 6 to 7 inches).   □   □   _____

19. If ordered, collect a sterile urine specimen. Hold the end of the catheter over the sterile specimen container and collect about 30 mL of urine. After collecting the specimen, pinch the catheter to stop the flow of urine. Move the specimen container aside and position the end of the catheter over the basin. Allow the rest of the urine to drain into the basin according to facility policy.   □   □   _____

20. Gently remove the catheter from the body. If the patient is an uncircumcised man, pull the foreskin back up over the head of the penis.   □   □   _____

21. Remove the sterile drapes and dispose of them in a facility-approved waste container.   □   □   _____

22. Remove your gloves and dispose of them in a facility-approved waste container.   □   □   _____

23. Adjust the person's hospital gown or pajama bottoms as necessary. Remove the bath blanket. Help the person back into a comfortable position, straighten the bottom linens, and draw the top linens over the person.   □   □   _____

24. Make sure that the bed is lowered to its lowest position and that the wheels are locked. If the side rails are in use, return the side rail to the raised position on the working side of the bed.   □   □   _____

25. Dispose of disposable items in a facility-approved waste container. Clean the equipment and return it to the area designated by your facility. If a specimen was collected, take the specimen container to the designated location.   □   □   _____

Finishing Up

26. Complete the "Finishing Up" steps.   □   □   _____

PROCEDURE 4-2
Inserting an Indwelling Urinary Catheter

	S	U	COMMENTS

Getting Ready

1. Complete the "Getting Ready" steps. ☐ ☐ _____

Procedure

2. Place the catheterization supplies on a clean surface, such as the bedside table. ☐ ☐ _____

3. Make sure that the bed is positioned at a comfortable working height (to promote good body mechanics) and that the wheels are locked. Lower the head of the bed to a flat position (as tolerated). If the side rails are in use, lower the side rail on the working side of the bed. The side rail on the opposite side of the bed should remain up. ☐ ☐ _____

4. Fanfold the linens to the foot of the bed. Position the person on his or her back. If the person is a woman, have her spread her legs apart and bend her knees slightly, if possible. (A woman can also be positioned on her side with her knees drawn to her chest.) Adjust the person's hospital gown or pajamas as necessary to expose the perineal area. Drape the person with the bath blanket. Position the bed protector under the person's buttocks to keep the bed linens dry. ☐ ☐ _____

5. Put on the non-sterile gloves and provide perineal care. ☐ ☐ _____

6. Dispose of the bed protector in a facility-approved waste container. Cover the perineal area, remove your gloves and dispose of them in a facility-approved waste container, and wash your hands. (If the side rails are in use, raise them before leaving the bedside.) ☐ ☐ _____

7. Return to the bedside. If the side rails are in use, lower the side rail on the working side of the bed. Expose the perineal area before creating the sterile field. ☐ ☐ _____

8. Using sterile technique, create the sterile field by opening the urinary catheter insertion kit on the work surface. (The paper wrapper becomes the sterile field.) ☐ ☐ _____

9. Remove the sterile glove package without touching the other items inside the urinary catheter insertion kit. Place the sterile glove package on the work surface next to the urinary catheter insertion kit. ☐ ☐ _____

10. **Position the first drape (the one without the opening).** Look for the edge of the sterile drape that is folded back to create a small area for you to grasp. Grasp the edge of the sterile drape with your thumb and index finger and lift the sterile drape straight up as you step back. Hold the sterile drape away from your body and allow it to unfold. Grasp the other top corner of the sterile drape with the thumb and index finger of your other hand and allow the sterile drape to unfold completely.

   a. Carefully fold the sterile drape in half lengthwise so that the sterile side is covering itself. ☐ ☐ _____

   b. Open the drape. The non-sterile side will be resting on your forearms. ☐ ☐ _____

   c. Ask the person to lift the buttocks. Position the sterile drape on the bed just under the buttocks with the sterile side facing up. Pull your arms out from under the sterile drape, being careful not to lean or reach over the sterile drape. ☐ ☐ _____

11. Put on the sterile gloves. ☐ ☐ _____

12. **Position the fenestrated drape (if used).** Look for the edge of the sterile drape that is folded back to create a small area for you to grasp. Grasp the edge of the sterile drape with your thumb and index finger and lift the sterile drape straight up as you step back. Hold the sterile drape away from your body and allow it to unfold. Grasp the other top corner of the sterile drape with the thumb and index finger of your other hand and allow the sterile drape to unfold completely.

   a. **Female patient:** Position the sterile drape over the perineum so that the labia are exposed, being careful not to touch anything but the fenestrated drape with your sterile gloves. ☐ ☐ _____

   b. **Male patient:** Position the sterile drape with the opening over the penis, being careful not to touch anything but the fenestrated drape with your sterile gloves. ☐ ☐ _____

13. Test the balloon on the catheter tip. Insert the tip of the prefilled syringe of sterile water in the injection port. Push the plunger to inject the water into the injection port.

   a. If the balloon inflates properly, withdraw the water by pulling back on the plunger. Leave the syringe attached to the injection port. ☐ ☐ _____

   b. If the balloon does not inflate properly or if you are unable to withdraw the water back into the syringe, obtain a new indwelling urinary catheter. ☐ ☐ _____

14. Pour antiseptic cleanser over the cotton balls or open the antiseptic cleansing swabs. ☐ ☐ _____

15. Open the packet of lubricant or uncap the lubricant syringe. Lubricate the tip of the catheter.
    a. **Female patient:** Lubricate 1 to 2 inches.
    b. **Male patient:** Lubricate 4 to 5 inches.
16. Clean the urinary meatus.
    a. **Female patient:** Spread the labia apart using your non-dominant hand. (Your non-dominant hand is now contaminated.) Using your dominant hand, pick up an antiseptic swab or use the forceps to pick up an antiseptic-soaked cotton ball. Using a clean cotton ball or swab for each stroke, first clean one side, then the other side, and finally the middle, starting at the top and stroking downward. To avoid contaminating the meatus, you must continue to hold the labia apart until the catheter insertion is finished.
    b. **Male patient:** Hold the penis using your non-dominant hand. (Your non-dominant hand is now contaminated.) Using your dominant hand, pick up an antiseptic swab or use the forceps to pick up an antiseptic-soaked cotton ball.
       • **If the man is circumcised:** Place the cotton ball or the antiseptic swab at the tip of the penis and stroke in a circular motion downward to the base of the penis. Repeat two more times using a clean cotton ball or swab for each stroke.
       • **If the man is uncircumcised:** Retract the foreskin by gently pushing the skin toward the base of the penis. Place the cotton ball or the antiseptic swab at the tip of the penis and stroke in a circular motion downward to the base of the penis. Repeat two more times using a clean cotton ball or swab for each stroke. To avoid contaminating the meatus, you must continue to retract the foreskin until the catheter insertion is finished.
17. Using your dominant hand, place the box holding the catheter between the person's legs. Avoid touching the bed, the linens, or the person with your sterile dominant hand.
18. Insert the urinary catheter. Pick up the catheter, holding it about 2 inches from the end. Leave the other end in the box.
    a. **Female patient:** Ask the patient to breathe deeply. Insert the catheter into the urinary meatus and advance it slowly until the catheter passes into the bladder and urine begins to flow (about 2 to 3 inches). Insert the catheter another 1 to 2 inches to ensure that the balloon passes into the bladder prior to inflation.

TIP: If you are catheterizing a woman and urine does not begin to flow, you probably inserted the catheter into the vaginal opening instead of the urinary meatus. (It is easy to confuse the vaginal opening and the urinary meatus, especially in older women.) Leave the catheter in place, obtain new supplies, and begin again. Leaving the first catheter in place will make it easier to identify the urinary meatus on your second attempt.

  b. **Male patient:** Ask the patient to breathe deeply. Insert the catheter into the urinary meatus and advance it slowly until the catheter passes into the bladder and urine begins to flow (about 6 to 7 inches). Continue to insert the catheter up to the bifurcation (fork) to ensure that the balloon passes into the bladder before inflation.

19. Inflate the balloon by injecting the sterile water into the injection port. Use all of the fluid in the syringe and then remove the syringe. If the person complains of pain, stop immediately and withdraw the water by pulling back on the plunger. (The balloon may be in the urethra instead of the bladder.) Remove the catheter and start over with new supplies.

20. Pull on the catheter gently until you meet resistance.

21. If the patient is an uncircumcised man, pull the foreskin back up over the head of the penis.

22. Loosely secure the catheter tubing to the person's body using the catheter strap or adhesive tape.

  a. **Female patient:** Secure the catheter tubing to the inner thigh.

  b. **Male patients:** Secure the catheter tubing to the inner thigh or lower abdomen.

23. Gently coil the remaining length of catheter tubing and secure it to the bed linens with a plastic clip or safety pin. Secure the urine drainage bag to the bed frame.

24. Remove the sterile drapes and dispose of them in a facility-approved waste container.

25. Remove your gloves and dispose of them in a facility-approved waste container.

26. Adjust the person's hospital gown or pajama bottoms as necessary. Remove the bath blanket. Help the person back into a comfortable position, straighten the bottom linens, and draw the top linens over the person.

27. Make sure that the bed is lowered to its lowest position and that the wheels are locked. If the side rails are in use, return the side rail to the raised position on the working side of the bed.

28. Dispose of disposable items in a facility-approved waste container. Clean the equipment and return it to the area designated by your facility. If a specimen was collected, take the specimen container to the designated location.

☐　☐　_____

Finishing Up

29. Complete the "Finishing Up" steps.

☐　☐　_____

PROCEDURE 4-3

Obtaining a Sterile Urine Specimen From a Patient With an Indwelling Urinary Catheter

Getting Ready

	S	U	COMMENTS
1. Complete the "Getting Ready" steps.	☐	☐	_____

Procedure

	S	U	COMMENTS
2. Place the supplies on a clean surface, such as the bed-side table. Complete the label with the person's name, room number, and other identifying information. Put the completed label on the specimen container. If the aspiration port is not "needle-less," attach the capped blunt needle to the 10-mL syringe.	☐	☐	_____
3. Make sure that the bed is positioned at a comfortable working height (to promote good body mechanics) and that the wheels are locked. If the side rails are in use, lower the side rail on the working side of the bed. The side rail on the opposite side of the bed should remain up.	☐	☐	_____
4. Fanfold the top linens to allow access to the aspiration port on the indwelling urinary catheter. Help the person to a comfortable position and adjust the person's hospital gown or pajamas as necessary to expose the aspiration port on the catheter. Remove the adhesive tape or catheter strap.	☐	☐	_____
5. Put on the gloves.	☐	☐	_____
6. Clamp the catheter tubing distal to the aspiration port.	☐	☐	_____
7. Allow urine to collect in the catheter tubing. (This may take 10 to 30 minutes.)	☐	☐	_____
8. Wipe the aspiration port with an alcohol wipe.	☐	☐	_____
9. If the aspiration port is not "needle-less," remove the cap from the needle and insert the needle and syringe into the aspiration port. If the aspiration port is "needle-less," attach the syringe to the aspiration port using a twisting motion. Withdraw 5 to 7 mL of urine by pulling back on the plunger.	☐	☐	_____
10. Remove the needle and syringe (or just the syringe if the aspiration port is "needle-less") from the aspiration port.	☐	☐	_____
11. Open the specimen container and place the lid on the over-bed table, with the inside of the lid facing up. Gently push the plunger to empty the urine into the specimen container. Avoid touching the inside of the specimen container with the needle and syringe or your hands.	☐	☐	_____
12. Discard the needle and syringe in a facility-approved sharps container.	☐	☐	_____

13. Unclamp the catheter tubing so the urine can flow into the urine drainage bag. ☐ ☐ _____

14. Put the lid on the specimen container. Make sure that the lid is tight. Place the specimen container into the transport bag. ☐ ☐ _____

15. Remove your gloves and dispose of them in a facility-approved waste container. Dispose of disposable items in a facility-approved waste container. ☐ ☐ _____

16. Loosely secure the catheter tubing to the person's body using the catheter strap or adhesive tape. ☐ ☐ _____

17. Adjust the person's hospital gown or pajama bottoms as necessary. Help the person back into a comfortable position, straighten the bottom linens, and draw the top linens over the person. ☐ ☐ _____

18. Make sure that the bed is lowered to its lowest position and that the wheels are locked. If the side rails are in use, return the side rail to the raised position on the working side of the bed. ☐ ☐ _____

19. Take the specimen container to the designated location. ☐ ☐ _____

Finishing Up

20. Complete the "Finishing Up" steps. ☐ ☐ _____

PROCEDURE 4-4

Irrigating an Indwelling Urinary Catheter Using Closed Irrigation

Getting Ready	S	U	COMMENTS
1. Complete the "Getting Ready" steps.	☐	☐	_____
2. Place the supplies on a clean surface, such as the bedside table.	☐	☐	_____
3. Put on the gloves. Empty the urine drainage bag and record the urine output according to facility policy. Empty and clean the graduate. Remove your gloves and dispose of them in a facility-approved waste container. Wash your hands.	☐	☐	_____
4. Make sure that the bed is positioned at a comfortable working height (to promote good body mechanics) and that the wheels are locked. If the side rails are in use, lower the side rail on the working side of the bed. The side rail on the opposite side of the bed should remain up.	☐	☐	_____
5. Fanfold the top linens to allow access to the aspiration port on the indwelling urinary catheter. Help the person to a comfortable position and adjust the person's hospital gown or pajamas as necessary to expose the aspiration port on the catheter. Remove the adhesive tape or catheter strap.	☐	☐	_____
6. Position the bed protector under the catheter and aspiration port to keep the linens dry.	☐	☐	_____
7. Using sterile technique, create the sterile field by opening the sterile basin on the work surface. (The basin becomes the sterile field.)	☐	☐	_____
8. Put on a clean pair of gloves.	☐	☐	_____
9. Fill the sterile basin with sterile irrigation fluid. Place the tip of the syringe in the sterile basin and withdraw irrigation fluid by pulling back on the plunger.	☐	☐	_____
10. If the aspiration port is not "needle-less," attach the capped blunt needle to the syringe.	☐	☐	_____
11. Wipe the aspiration port with an alcohol wipe.	☐	☐	_____
12. Clamp the catheter tubing distal to the aspiration port.	☐	☐	_____
13. If the aspiration port is not "needle-less," remove the cap from the needle and insert the needle and syringe into the aspiration port. If the aspiration port is "needle-less," attach the syringe to the aspiration port using a twisting motion. Push the plunger to inject the irrigation fluid into the aspiration port. Repeat as many times as ordered or necessary.	☐	☐	_____
14. Discard the needle and syringe in a facility-approved sharps container.	☐	☐	_____

15. Unclamp the catheter tubing so that the urine can flow into the urine drainage bag.

   ☐ ☐ _____

16. Remove your gloves and dispose of them in a facility-approved waste container. Dispose of disposable items in a facility-approved waste container.

   ☐ ☐ _____

17. Loosely secure the catheter tubing to the person's body using the catheter strap or adhesive tape.

   ☐ ☐ _____

18. Adjust the person's hospital gown or pajama bottoms as necessary. Remove the bed protector. Help the person back into a comfortable position, straighten the bottom linens, and draw the top linens over the person.

   ☐ ☐ _____

19. Make sure that the bed is lowered to its lowest position and that the wheels are locked. If the side rails are in use, return the side rail to the raised position on the working side of the bed.

   ☐ ☐ _____

Finishing Up

20. Complete the "Finishing Up" steps.

   ☐ ☐ _____

PROCEDURE 4-5
Removing an Indwelling Urinary Catheter

	S	U	COMMENTS

Getting Ready

1. Complete the "Getting Ready" steps. ☐ ☐ _____

Procedure

2. Place the supplies on a clean surface, such as the bed-side table. ☐ ☐ _____

3. Put on the gloves. Empty the urine drainage bag and record the urine output according to facility policy. Empty and clean the graduate. Remove your gloves and dispose of them in a facility-approved waste container. Wash your hands. ☐ ☐ _____

4. Make sure that the bed is positioned at a comfortable working height (to promote good body mechanics) and that the wheels are locked. Lower the head of the bed to a flat position (as tolerated). If the side rails are in use, lower the side rail on the working side of the bed. The side rail on the opposite side of the bed should remain up. ☐ ☐ _____

5. Fanfold the top linens to the foot of the bed. Position the person on his or her back. If the person is a woman, have her spread her legs apart and bend her knees slightly, if possible. (A woman can also be positioned on her side with her knees drawn to her chest.) Adjust the person's hospital gown or pajamas as necessary to expose the perineal area. Drape the person with the bath blanket. Position the bed protector under the person's buttocks to keep the bed linens dry. ☐ ☐ _____

6. Remove the adhesive tape or catheter strap. ☐ ☐ _____

7. Put on a clean pair of gloves. ☐ ☐ _____

8. Deflate the balloon on the catheter tip: Insert the tip of the syringe in the injection port. Withdraw the water in the balloon by pulling back on the plunger. Make sure to withdraw all of the water (remember that some balloons hold up to 30 mL of water). ☐ ☐ _____

9. Gently pull the catheter out of the bladder. If the person experiences pain or if there is resistance, stop and make sure that the balloon is completely deflated. If the balloon is completely deflated but the person is still experiencing pain or there is resistance, call for the nurse. ☐ ☐ _____

10. Discard the catheter, syringe, catheter tubing, and urine drainage bag in a facility-approved waste container. ☐ ☐ _____

11. Provide perineal care. Remove your gloves and dispose of them in a facility-approved waste container. Wash your hands.

12. Adjust the person's hospital gown or pajama bottoms as necessary. Remove the bed protector. Help the person back into a comfortable position, straighten the bottom linens, and draw the top linens over the person.

13. Make sure that the bed is lowered to its lowest position and that the wheels are locked. If the side rails are in use, return the side rail to the raised position on the working side of the bed.

Finishing Up

14. Complete the "Finishing Up" steps.

CHAPTER 5 PROCEDURE CHECKLISTS

PROCEDURE 5-1
Removing a Nasogastric Tube

	S	U	COMMENTS

Getting Ready

1. Complete the "Getting Ready" steps. ☐ ☐ _____

Procedure

2. Make sure that the bed is positioned at a comfortable working height (to promote good body mechanics) and that the wheels are locked. If the side rails are in use, lower the side rail on the working side of the bed. The side rail on the opposite side of the bed should remain up. Raise the head of the bed to the semi-Fowler's or Fowler's position. ☐ ☐ _____

3. Place the disposable bed protector across the person's chest. Have the emesis basin nearby in case the person gags or vomits. ☐ ☐ _____

4. Put on the gloves. ☐ ☐ _____

5. Unpin the tube from the person's gown and remove the tape from the person's nose. ☐ ☐ _____

6. Ask the person to take a deep breath and hold it while you pull out the nasogastric tube. (Holding the breath prevents the person from inhaling as the tube is pulled out. If the person inhales as the tube is being pulled out, stomach contents could be aspirated into the lungs.) Pull out the tube in one continuous motion. ☐ ☐ _____

7. Dispose of the nasogastric tube in a facility-approved waste container. ☐ ☐ _____

8. Offer tissues to the person so that she can blow her nose, if desired. Assist the person with oral care. ☐ ☐ _____

9. Remove your gloves and dispose of them in a facility-approved waste container. ☐ ☐ _____

10. If the side rails are in use, return them to the raised position. Lower the head of the bed as the person requests. Make sure that the bed is lowered to its lowest position and that the wheels are locked. ☐ ☐ _____

Finishing Up

11. Complete the "Finishing Up" steps. ☐ ☐ _____

PROCEDURE 5-2
Monitoring the Blood Glucose Level

Getting Ready	S	U	COMMENTS
1. Complete the "Getting Ready" steps.	☐	☐	_____

Procedure

	S	U	COMMENTS
2. Put on the gloves.	☐	☐	_____
3. Help the person to wash his hands with the soap and water. Dry the person's hands with the towel.	☐	☐	_____
4. Turn the blood glucose meter on and wait until the "ready" sign appears on the display screen.	☐	☐	_____
5. Remove a testing strip from the bottle. Immediately replace the cap on the bottle. Make sure that the code on the testing strip matches the code on the blood glucose meter. Depending on the type of blood glucose meter you are using, you may be required to insert the testing strip into the meter now.	☐	☐	_____
6. Prepare the lancet by removing the safety cap. Grasp the person's finger and hold the lancet at a 90-degree angle to the skin. (Try to avoid the middle of the finger pad because this area has the highest concentration of nerve endings.) Press the lancet straight down to pierce the person's skin.	☐	☐	_____
7. Gently squeeze the site until a drop of blood forms.	☐	☐	_____
8. Transfer the drop of blood from the person's finger to the testing strip by gently rolling the person's finger over the testing strip or by gently touching the person's finger to the testing strip. Make sure to apply an adequate amount of blood to the testing strip, but not too much.	☐	☐	_____
9. If the testing strip is not already in the blood glucose meter, insert the testing strip into the blood glucose meter, according to the manufacturer's instructions.	☐	☐	_____
10. Apply pressure to the puncture site using tissue or a cotton ball.	☐	☐	_____
11. Record the reading on the blood glucose meter. Turn off the blood glucose meter if it does not automatically turn itself off.	☐	☐	_____
12. Dispose of the lancet in a sharps container. Dispose of the test strip in a facility-approved waste container.	☐	☐	_____
13. Remove your gloves and dispose of them according to facility policy. Wash your hands.	☐	☐	_____

Finishing Up

	S	U	COMMENTS
14. Complete the "Finishing Up" steps.	☐	☐	_____

CHAPTER 6 PROCEDURE CHECKLISTS

PROCEDURE 6-1
Providing Tracheostomy Site Care

Getting Ready	S	U	COMMENTS
1. Complete the "Getting Ready" steps.	☐	☐	_____
2. Make sure that the bed is positioned at a comfortable working height (to promote good body mechanics) and that the wheels are locked. If the side rails are in use, lower the side rail on the working side of the bed. The side rail on the opposite side of the bed should remain up. Raise the head of the bed to the semi-Fowler's or Fowler's position.	☐	☐	
3. Put on the gloves.	☐	☐	_____
4. Remove the soiled dressing by sliding it out from underneath the faceplate. Dispose of the soiled dressing in a facility-approved waste container.	☐	☐	_____
5. Remove your gloves and dispose of them in a facility-approved waste container. Wash your hands.	☐	☐	_____
6. Remove one of the sterile basins from its package, being careful not to touch the inside of the basin. Pour sterile saline or sterile water into the sterile basin.	☐	☐	_____
7. Put on a clean pair of gloves.	☐	☐	_____
8. Dip a cotton-tipped applicator or a gauze sponge into the sterile saline or sterile water. Gently lift up the faceplate and clean the skin around the tracheostomy by placing the moistened cotton-tipped applicator or gauze sponge next to the tracheostomy tube and moving it in a circular motion around the tracheostomy tube. Move outward from the tracheostomy tube using a clean moistened cotton-tipped applicator or gauze sponge for each stroke.	☐	☐	_____
9. Pat the skin dry with a sterile gauze sponge.	☐	☐	_____
10. Slide the clean tracheostomy dressing under the faceplate.	☐	☐	_____
11. Change the tracheostomy ties:			
a. Take a piece of tracheostomy tie approximately 18 to 24 inches long. Trim the ends of the tie on the diagonal.	☐	☐	_____
b. Insert one end of the tie through the opening on the faceplate next to the old tie. Pull the end of the new tie until the ends are even.	☐	☐	_____

c. Bring both ends of the new tie behind the person's neck and insert one end through the opening on the faceplate on the other side. Tie the ends of the tie in a double square knot. Make sure the tie is snug but not too tight. You should be able to slide your finger between the tie and the person's neck.

☐ ☐ _____

d. Carefully remove the old tie by untying it or cutting it.

☐ ☐ _____

12. Remove your gloves and dispose of them in a facility-approved waste container.

☐ ☐ _____

13. If the side rails are in use, return them to the raised position. Lower the head of the bed as the person requests. Make sure that the bed is lowered to its lowest position and that the wheels are locked.

☐ ☐ _____

14. Dispose of disposable items in a facility-approved waste container.

☐ ☐ _____

Finishing Up

15. Complete the "Finishing Up" steps.

☐ ☐ _____

CHAPTER 7 PROCEDURE CHECKLISTS

PROCEDURE 7-1
Performing Venipuncture Using a Vacuum Tube System

	S	U	COMMENTS

Getting Ready

1. Complete the "Getting Ready" steps. ☐ ☐ _____

Procedure

2. Place the venipuncture supplies on a clean surface. Place the needle in the tube holder. Make sure the vacuum tubes are within easy reach. Fold down the top edges of the plastic bag to make a cuff. Place the cuffed bag within easy reach. ☐ ☐ _____

3. Make sure that the bed is positioned at a comfortable working height (to promote good body mechanics) and that the wheels are locked. If the side rails are in use, lower the side rail on the working side. The side rail on the opposite side of the bed should remain up. ☐ ☐ _____

4. Assist the person to a seated or supine position. The person's arm should be fully extended, pointed slightly downward, and supported by a firm surface. If necessary, roll up the person's sleeve to expose the antecubital space. ☐ ☐ _____

5. Select a vein: Apply the tourniquet 3 to 6 inches above the site where you are planning to insert the needle (see Fig. 7-6). Ask the person to make a fist. Identify a vein that is suitable for venipuncture. Release the tourniquet. ☐ ☐ _____

6. Put on the gloves. ☐ ☐ _____

7. Clean the site where you are planning to insert the needle.

   a. **Alcohol or Betadine swabs:** Place the swab on the intended insertion site and move it outward in a circular motion. If using Betadine, allow the area to dry for 60 seconds. ☐ ☐ _____

   b. **Chlorhexidine:** Place the swab on the intended insertion site and scrub using a back-and-forth motion for at least 30 seconds. Allow the area to dry for 30 seconds. ☐ ☐ _____

8. Reapply the tourniquet 3 to 6 inches above the site where you intend to insert the needle. ☐ ☐ _____

9. Hold the tube holder in your dominant hand. Remove the needle cover by pulling it straight off. ☐ ☐ _____

10. Place the thumb of your non-dominant hand below the site where you intend to insert the needle and pull down so that the skin over the insertion site is stretched tight. ☐ ☐ _____

11. If necessary, ask the person to make a fist again. Let the person know that you are about to insert the needle and tell the person to expect to feel a "pinch." With the bevel of the needle facing up and at a 15- to 30-degree angle to the skin, insert the needle into the vein. ☐ ☐ _____

12. Place the first vacuum tube into the tube holder. Use your index and middle fingers to stabilize the tube holder as you use your thumb to push the vacuum tube onto the needle. ☐ ☐ _____

13. Let the vacuum tube fill until the vacuum runs out and the blood stops flowing. When the blood stops flowing, remove the vacuum tube from the tube holder, making sure to stabilize the tube holder to minimize movement of the needle. If the vacuum tube contains an additive, gently turn the tube upside down and then right side up a few times to mix the additive and the blood specimen. ☐ ☐ _____

14. Repeat steps 12 and 13 until all of the ordered blood specimens have been obtained. Release the tourniquet just before the last vacuum tube finishes filling. ☐ ☐ _____

15. Gently hold a gauze pad over the needle insertion site. Remove the needle from the vein by pulling it straight out. ☐ ☐ _____

16. Hold the gauze pad in place, applying pressure for 2 to 3 minutes. Place the gauze pad in the cuffed plastic bag. ☐ ☐ _____

17. Open the adhesive bandage and apply it to the needle insertion site. ☐ ☐ _____

18. Dispose of the tube holder and needle in a facility-approved sharps container. ☐ ☐ _____

19. Complete the specimen labels according to facility policy. Apply the labels to the tubes per facility policy. Place the tubes in a plastic transport bag (if required at your facility). ☐ ☐ _____

20. Remove your gloves and dispose of them in a facility-approved waste container. ☐ ☐ _____

21. Check to make sure that the bleeding has stopped. Adjust the person's clothing as necessary. Help the person back into a comfortable position, straighten the bottom linens, and draw the top linens over the person. ☐ ☐ _____

22. Make sure that the bed is lowered to its lowest position and that the wheels are locked. If the side rails are in use, return the side rail to the raised position on the working side of the bed. ☐ ☐ _____

23. Dispose of disposable items in a facility-approved
    waste container. Clean the equipment and return it
    to the area designated by your facility. Take the
    blood specimens to the designated location.

Finishing Up

24. Complete the "Finishing Up" steps.

PROCEDURE 7-2
Removing a Peripheral Line

Getting Ready	S	U	COMMENTS
1. Complete the "Getting Ready" steps.	☐	☐	_____

Procedure

	S	U	COMMENTS
2. Place the supplies on a clean surface. Fold down the top edges of the plastic bag to make a cuff. Place the cuffed bag within easy reach.	☐	☐	_____
3. Check the clamp to verify that the nurse has stopped the flow of fluids through the peripheral line.	☐	☐	_____
4. Make sure that the bed is positioned at a comfortable working height (to promote good body mechanics) and that the wheels are locked. If the side rails are in use, lower the side rail on the working side. The side rail on the opposite side of the bed should remain up.	☐	☐	_____
5. Help the person to a comfortable position that allows access to the insertion site. If necessary, roll up the person's sleeve to expose the insertion site.	☐	☐	_____
6. Put on the gloves.	☐	☐	_____
7. Remove the adhesive dressing covering the insertion site carefully using a peeling action. Place the soiled dressing in the cuffed plastic bag.	☐	☐	_____
8. Gently hold a gauze pad over the insertion site. Remove the catheter from the vein by pulling it straight out.	☐	☐	_____
9. Hold the gauze pad in place, applying pressure for 2 to 3 minutes. Place the gauze pad in the cuffed plastic bag.	☐	☐	_____
10. Observe the end of the catheter to make sure the entire catheter was removed.			
a. If the catheter looks damaged, call the nurse to the room immediately.	☐	☐	_____
b. If no problems are noted, dispose of the catheter in a facility-approved sharps container.	☐	☐	_____
11. Clean the insertion site.			
a. **Alcohol or Betadine swabs:** Place the swab on the insertion site and move it outward in a circular motion. If using Betadine, allow the area to dry for 60 seconds.	☐	☐	_____
b. **Chlorhexidine:** Place the swab on the insertion site and scrub using a back-and-forth motion for at least 30 seconds. Allow the area to dry for 30 seconds.	☐	☐	_____
12. Open the adhesive bandage and apply it to the insertion site.	☐	☐	_____

13. Remove your gloves and dispose of them in a facility-approved waste container. ☐ ☐ _____

14. Check to make sure that the bleeding has stopped. Adjust the person's clothing as necessary. Help the person back into a comfortable position, straighten the bottom linens, and draw the top linens over the person. ☐ ☐ _____

15. Make sure that the bed is lowered to its lowest position and that the wheels are locked. If the side rails are in use, return the side rail to the raised position on the working side of the bed. ☐ ☐ _____

16. Dispose of disposable items in a facility-approved waste container. Clean the equipment and return it to the area designated by your facility. ☐ ☐ _____

Finishing Up

17. Complete the "Finishing Up" steps. ☐ ☐ _____

CHAPTER 8 PROCEDURE CHECKLISTS

PROCEDURE 8-1
Setting Up Continuous Cardiac Monitoring

	S	U	COMMENTS

Getting Ready

1. Complete the "Getting Ready" steps. ☐ ☐ _____

Procedure

2. Prepare the equipment.
   a. **Hardwire:** Place the monitor close to the person's bed, plug in the power cord, and turn on the monitor. Insert the cable into the appropriate socket in the monitor and connect the lead wires to the cable if necessary. (In some systems, the lead wires and cable are kept connected to the monitors.) ☐ ☐ _____

   b. **Telemetry:** Insert a new or freshly charged battery into the transmitter box. Check to make sure the battery works by turning on the device. ☐ ☐ _____

3. Make sure the bed is positioned at a comfortable working height (to promote good body mechanics) and that the wheels are locked. If the side rails are in use, lower the side rail on the working side of the bed. The side rail on the opposite side of the bed should remain up. ☐ ☐ _____

4. Fanfold the top linens to below the person's waist. Adjust the person's clothing as necessary to expose the chest. (If the person is a woman, use the bath towel to cover the breasts for modesty.) ☐ ☐ _____

5. Determine the correct position for each electrode according to the system in use (see Box 8-2). Make sure that the skin in the areas where the electrodes will be applied is free from irritation, bruising, and breaks. If the person's chest is excessively hairy, use the clippers to remove the hair in the areas where the electrodes will be placed. ☐ ☐ _____

6. Clean each area where an electrode will be placed with an alcohol pad to remove skin oils that may interfere with electrode function or adhesion. Dry each area with a gauze pad. ☐ ☐ _____

7. Peel off the backing of the electrode and check to make sure the gel is moist. If the gel is dry, the electrode should be discarded. ☐ ☐ _____

8. Apply the electrode, pressing it down firmly to ensure a good seal. Repeat steps 7 and 8 until all of the electrodes have been applied. ☐ ☐ _____

9. Snap the lead wires to the appropriate electrodes.

   a. **Three-electrode system:** RA = white, LA = black, LL = red ☐ ☐ _____

   b. **Five-electrode system:** RA = white, RL = green, LA = black, LL = red, C = brown ☐ ☐ _____

10. Check to make sure the lead wires are attached securely to the electrodes. Observe the ECG waveforms on the monitor. Adjust the monitor or the position of the electrodes as needed to obtain a clear tracing. ☐ ☐ _____

11. Set the alarm rate limits according to your facility's policy or as ordered by the doctor. Turn on the alarm. ☐ ☐ _____

12. Adjust the person's clothing as necessary to cover the chest. If using a telemetry monitoring system, place the transmitter box in the carrying pouch. Secure the pouch to the person (either by placing the pouch around the person's neck or securing it to the person's clothing). ☐ ☐ _____

13. Straighten the bottom linens and draw the top linens over the person. Make sure that the bed is lowered to its lowest position and that the wheels are locked. If the side rails are in use, return them to the raised position. ☐ ☐ _____

14. Record a rhythm strip and label it with the person's name and room number, the date, and the time according to your facility's policy. Place the rhythm strip in the person's chart. ☐ ☐ _____

Finishing Up

15. Complete the "Finishing Up" steps. ☐ ☐ _____

PROCEDURE 8-2
Obtaining a 12-Lead Electrocardiograph

	S	U	COMMENTS

Getting Ready

1. Complete the "Getting Ready" steps. ☐ ☐ _____

Procedure

2. Place the electrocardiograph close to the person's bed, plug in the power cord, and turn the electrocardiograph on. If necessary, enter the required patient information into the machine. Check to make sure that there is enough paper and replace the roll of paper if necessary. ☐ ☐ _____

3. Make sure the bed is positioned at a comfortable working height (to promote good body mechanics) and that the wheels are locked. If the side rails are in use, lower the side rail on the working side of the bed. The side rail on the opposite side of the bed should remain up. Lower the head of the bed so that the bed is flat (as tolerated). ☐ ☐ _____

4. Position the person in the supine position in the center of the bed with the arms out to the sides. Make sure that the person's feet are not touching the footboard of the bed. ☐ ☐ _____

5. Spread the bath blanket over the top linens (and the person). If the person is able, have him hold the bath blanket. If not, tuck the corners under the person's shoulders. Fanfold the top linens to the foot of the bed. Adjust the person's clothing as necessary to expose the chest, arms, and legs. ☐ ☐ _____

6. Fold the bath blanket down to expose the chest and arms and up from the bottom to expose the person's lower legs. (If the person is a woman, use the bath towel to cover the breasts for modesty.) ☐ ☐ _____

7. Apply the limb electrodes and leads.

   a. Determine the correct position for each electrode. When selecting sites for the limb electrodes, choose sites that are fleshy rather than muscular or bony. Make sure that the skin in the areas where the electrodes will be applied is free from irritation, bruising, and breaks. If the person's limbs are excessively hairy, use the clippers to remove the hair in the areas where the electrodes will be placed. ☐ ☐ _____

   b. Clean each area where an electrode will be placed with an alcohol pad to remove skin oils that may interfere with electrode function or adhesion. Dry each area with a gauze pad. ☐ ☐ _____

   c. Peel off the backing of the electrode and check to make sure the gel is moist. If the gel is dry, the electrode should be discarded. ☐ ☐ _____

   d. Apply the electrode, pressing it down firmly to ensure a good seal. Repeat steps 7c and 7d until all of the limb electrodes have been applied. ☐ ☐ _____

   e. Snap the lead wires to the appropriate electrodes: RA = white, RL = green, LA = black, LL = red. ☐ ☐ _____

8. Apply the chest electrodes and leads. If the person is a woman, move the bath towel to expose the breasts as necessary. You will need to lift the breasts and place the electrodes below the breast tissue on the chest wall.

   a. Determine the correct position for each electrode (see Box 8-1). Make sure that the skin in the areas where the electrodes will be applied is free from irritation, bruising, and breaks. If the person's chest is excessively hairy, use the clippers to remove the hair in the areas where the electrodes will be placed. ☐ ☐ _____

   b. Clean each area where an electrode will be placed with an alcohol pad to remove skin oils that may interfere with electrode function or adhesion. Dry each area with a gauze pad. ☐ ☐ _____

   c. Peel off the backing of the electrode and check to make sure the gel is moist. If the gel is dry, the electrode should be discarded. ☐ ☐ _____

   d. Apply the electrode, pressing it down firmly to ensure a good seal. Repeat steps 8c and 8d until all of the chest electrodes have been applied. ☐ ☐ _____

   e. Snap the lead wires to the appropriate electrodes (V_1 through V_6 = brown). ☐ ☐ _____

9. Ask the person to relax and breathe normally. Remind the person to lie still and not talk during the ECG recording. Let the person know that the ECG recording will only take a few minutes. ☐ ☐ _____

10. Press the button that starts the recording. ☐ ☐ _____

11. Check the ECG tracings on the recording paper to make sure that all of the leads recorded clearly. If the ECG tracings are not clear, it may be because an electrode or lead wire became loose during the recording. If the first recording is not clear, check all of the electrodes and lead wires and re-run the ECG recording. ☐ ☐ _____

12. Remove the electrodes and clean the person's skin if necessary. Adjust the person's clothing as necessary to cover the chest, arms, and legs. ☐ ☐ _____

13. Straighten the bottom linens and draw the top linens over the person. Remove the bath blanket from underneath the top linens. Make sure that the bed is lowered to its lowest position and that the wheels are locked. If the side rails are in use, return them to the raised position. Raise the head of the bed, as the person requests.   □   □   _____

14. Label the ECG with the person's name and room number, the date, and the time according to your facility's policy, if the machine did not do it automatically. Place the ECG in the person's chart or other designated place per your facility's policy.   □   □   _____

15. Gather the soiled linens and place them in the linen hamper or linen bag. Dispose of disposable items in a facility-approved waste container. Clean the equipment and return it to the storage area.   □   □   _____

Finishing Up

16. Complete the "Finishing Up" steps.   □   □   _____

CHAPTER 14 PROCEDURE CHECKLISTS

PROCEDURE 14-1
Administering Oral Medications

Getting Ready	S	U	COMMENTS
1. Wash your hands.	☐	☐	_____
2. Gather your supplies: non-sterile gloves (if splitting or crushing tablets), medication administration record (MAR) or medication order, medication cup (paper for tablets or capsules; plastic for liquids), pill splitter or medication-crushing device, if needed, paper cup	☐	☐	_____

Procedure

	S	U	COMMENTS
3. In the medication room, select the ordered medication from the medication cart or computer-operated drawer system. Make sure the name of the medication on the medication label is the same as the name of the medication on the MAR or medication order.	☐	☐	_____
4. Check the route of administration and the dose on the MAR or medication order.	☐	☐	_____
5. Measure the amount of medication you need.			
a. **Tablets:** Dispense the number of tablets you need into the medication cup.	☐	☐	_____
• **To split a tablet:** If you must split a tablet to achieve the proper dose, use a pill splitter. Put on the gloves and place the tablet in the pill splitter. After splitting the pill, place half of the tablet in the medication cup and return the other half to the medicine bottle or discard it, according to facility policy. Remove your gloves.			
• **To crush a tablet:** If the MAR or medication order states that the tablet is to be crushed, put on the gloves and place the tablet in the medication-crushing device. Crush the tablet into a fine powder. Place the powder in the medication cup. Remove your gloves.			
b. **Capsules:** Dispense the number of capsules that you need into the medication cup.	☐	☐	_____
c. **Liquids:** Place the medication cup at eye level on a level surface. Pour the liquid into the medication cup until the liquid reaches the measurement marking on the side of the cup that corresponds with the ordered dose.	☐	☐	_____
6. Repeat steps 3 through 5 for each of the medications ordered for the person on the MAR or medication order.	☐	☐	_____

7. Compare the medications you have prepared to the MAR or medication order to make sure you have the correct medications in the correct doses. Recheck the patient's or resident's name on the MAR or medication order.   ☐ ☐ _____

8. Take the medications to the person.   ☐ ☐ _____

9. Identify the person by having him state his name while you check his identification band.   ☐ ☐ _____

10. Explain the procedure.   ☐ ☐ _____

11. Fill the paper cup with water from the bedside pitcher.   ☐ ☐ _____

12. Administer the medication.

   a. Hand the cup of water and the medication cup containing the medication to the person.   ☐ ☐ _____

   b. Stay with the person while he takes the medication. It is important to make sure that the person swallows the medication, and to be available to assist in case the person chokes. If the person drops a tablet or capsule, it must be discarded and replaced.   ☐ ☐ _____

13. Dispose of disposable items in a facility-approved waste container. Clean the equipment and return it to the storage area.   ☐ ☐ _____

Finishing Up

14. Complete the "Finishing Up" steps.   ☐ ☐ _____

PROCEDURE 14-2
Administering a Transdermal Patch

Getting Ready	S	U	COMMENTS
1. Wash your hands.	☐	☐	_____
2. Gather your supplies: gloves, paper towels, medication administration record (MAR) or medication order, wash basin, soap, washcloth, towel	☐	☐	_____

Procedure

	S	U	COMMENTS
3. In the medication room, select the ordered medication from the medication cart or computer-operated drawer system. Make sure the name of the medication on the medication label is the same as the name of the medication on the MAR or medication order.	☐	☐	_____
4. Check the route of administration and the dose on the MAR or medication order. Recheck the patient's or resident's name on the MAR or medication order.	☐	☐	_____
5. Take the medications to the person.	☐	☐	_____
6. Identify the person by having her state her name while you check her identification band.	☐	☐	_____
7. Explain the procedure.	☐	☐	_____
8. Cover the over-bed table with paper towels. Place the supplies on the over-bed table.	☐	☐	_____
9. Make sure the bed is positioned at a comfortable working height (to promote good body mechanics) and that the wheels are locked.	☐	☐	_____
10. Fill the wash basin with warm water (110°F [43.3°C] to 115°F [46.1°C] on the bath thermometer). Place the basin on the over-bed table.	☐	☐	_____
11. Put on the gloves.	☐	☐	_____
12. Expose the area where the old transdermal patch is located. Gently remove the old transdermal patch and dispose of it in a facility-approved waste container.	☐	☐	_____
13. Wash, rinse, and dry the area where the old patch was located.	☐	☐	_____
14. Cover the area where the old transdermal patch was located and expose the area where the new transdermal patch is to be placed.	☐	☐	_____
15. Write your initials, the date, and the time on the transdermal patch.	☐	☐	_____
16. Remove the backing from the new transdermal patch, being careful not to touch the adhesive side.	☐	☐	_____
17. Place the transdermal patch on the person's skin, pressing firmly.	☐	☐	_____

18. Remove your gloves and dispose of them in a facility-approved waste container.
☐ ☐ _____

19. Dispose of disposable items in a facility-approved waste container. Clean the equipment and return it to the storage area.
☐ ☐ _____

Finishing Up

20. Complete the "Finishing Up" steps.
☐ ☐ _____

PROCEDURE 14-3
Administering Eye Drops

Getting Ready	S	U	COMMENTS
1. Wash your hands.	☐	☐	_____
2. Gather your supplies: gloves, medication administration record (MAR) or medication order, washcloth, saline solution, tissues	☐	☐	_____

Procedure	S	U	COMMENTS
3. In the medication room, select the ordered medication from the medication cart or computer-operated drawer system. Make sure the name of the medication on the medication label is the same as the name of the medication on the MAR or medication order.	☐	☐	_____
4. Check the route of administration and the dose on the MAR or medication order. Recheck the patient's or resident's name on the MAR or medication order.	☐	☐	_____
5. Take the medications to the person.	☐	☐	_____
6. Identify the person by having her state her name while you check her identification band.	☐	☐	_____
7. Explain the procedure.	☐	☐	_____
8. Put on the gloves.	☐	☐	_____
9. Moisten the washcloth with the saline solution and wash the person's eye, moving from the inside corner to the outside corner. Use a different part of the washcloth for each eye.	☐	☐	_____
10. Help the person tilt her head back.	☐	☐	_____
11. Remove the cap from the medication bottle.	☐	☐	_____
12. Place two fingers or your thumb below the person's eye and gently pull the skin down to expose the lower conjunctival sac.	☐	☐	_____
13. Ask the person to look upward. Turn the medication bottle upside down and squeeze the required number of drops into the lower conjunctival sac. Avoid touching the tip of the dropper to the person's eye.	☐	☐	_____
14. Release the skin to allow the lower eyelid to return to its normal position. Ask the person to close her eyes. Offer the person a tissue to blot drainage but remind her not to rub the eye.	☐	☐	_____
15. Replace the cap on the medication bottle.	☐	☐	_____
16. Remove your gloves and dispose of them in a facility-approved waste container.	☐	☐	_____

17. Dispose of disposable items in a facility-approved waste container. Clean the equipment and return it to the storage area.

☐ ☐ _____

Finishing Up

18. Complete the "Finishing Up" steps.

☐ ☐ _____

PROCEDURE 14-4
Administering Ear Drops

	S	U	COMMENTS
Getting Ready			
1. Wash your hands.	☐	☐	_____
2. Gather your supplies: medication administration record (MAR) or medication order, washcloth, saline solution, tissues, cotton ball (if ordered)	☐	☐	_____

Procedure

	S	U	COMMENTS
3. In the medication room, select the ordered medication from the medication cart or computer-operated drawer system. Make sure the name of the medication on the medication label is the same as the name of the medication on the MAR or medication order.	☐	☐	_____
4. Check the route of administration and the dose on the MAR or medication order. Recheck the patient's or resident's name on the MAR or medication order.	☐	☐	_____
5. Take the medications to the person.	☐	☐	_____
6. Identify the person by having him state his name while you check his identification band.	☐	☐	_____
7. Explain the procedure.	☐	☐	_____
8. Position the person:			
a. If the person cannot sit up, help him into the lateral position so the affected ear is facing up.	☐	☐	_____
b. If the person can sit up, help him tilt his head to the side so the affected ear is facing up.	☐	☐	_____
9. Moisten the washcloth with the saline solution and wash the person's outer ear.	☐	☐	_____
10. Remove the cap from the medication bottle.	☐	☐	_____
11. To straighten the ear canal, grasp the top portion of the person's ear and gently pull:			
a. Up and back (in an adult)	☐	☐	_____
b. Straight back (in a child)	☐	☐	_____
12. Turn the medication bottle upside down and squeeze the required number of drops into the ear canal. Avoid touching the tip of the dropper to the person's ear.	☐	☐	_____
13. Release the ear. Ask the person to remain in the lateral position or with the head turned to the side for several minutes to prevent the medication from running out of the ear. Gently rubbing the area where the ear meets the cheek bone may help move the medication to where it is needed.	☐	☐	_____
14. If ordered, place a cotton ball in the opening of the ear to catch any drainage.	☐	☐	_____

15. Replace the cap on the medication bottle.   ☐ ☐   _____
16. Dispose of disposable items in a facility-approved   ☐ ☐   _____
    waste container. Clean the equipment and return it
    to the storage area.

Finishing Up

17. Complete the "Finishing Up" steps.   ☐ ☐   _____

PROCEDURE 14-5
Administering a Rectal Suppository

	S	U	COMMENTS
Getting Ready			
1. Wash your hands.	☐	☐	_____
2. Gather your supplies: medication administration record (MAR) or medication order, non-sterile gloves, lubricant jelly, tissues, bath blanket	☐	☐	_____
Procedure			
3. In the medication room, select the ordered medication from the medication cart or computer-operated drawer system. Make sure the name of the medication on the medication label is the same as the name of the medication on the MAR or medication order.	☐	☐	_____
4. Check the route of administration and the dose on the MAR or medication order. Recheck the patient's or resident's name on the MAR or medication order.	☐	☐	_____
5. Take the medications to the person.	☐	☐	_____
6. Identify the person by having him state his name while you check his identification band.	☐	☐	_____
7. Explain the procedure.	☐	☐	_____
8. Make sure that the bed is positioned at a comfortable working height (to promote good body mechanics) and that the wheels are locked.	☐	☐	_____
9. If the side rails are in use, lower the side rail on the working side of the bed. The side rail on the opposite side of the bed should remain up. Lower the head of the bed so that the bed is flat (as tolerated).	☐	☐	_____
10. Spread the bath blanket over the top linens and the person. If the person is able, have him hold a bath blanket. If not, tuck the corners under his shoulders. Fanfold the top linens to the foot of the bed.	☐	☐	_____
11. Ask the person to lie on his left side, facing away from you, in Sims' position. Help him into this position if necessary.	☐	☐	_____
12. Put on the gloves.	☐	☐	_____
13. Adjust the bath blanket and the person's hospital gown or pajama bottoms as necessary to expose the person's buttocks.	☐	☐	_____
14. Remove the suppository from its package. Open the lubricant package and apply a small amount of lubricant to the rounded end of the suppository.	☐	☐	_____

15. With one hand, raise the person's upper buttock to expose the anus. Using your other hand, gently and carefully insert the suppository into the person's rectum (not more than 3 to 4 inches for adults). Never force the suppository into the rectum. If you are unable to insert the suppository, stop and call the nurse. ☐ ☐ _____

16. Wipe the person's anal area with a tissue to remove the lubricant and adjust the person's hospital gown or pajama bottoms as necessary to cover the buttocks. ☐ ☐ _____

17. Remove your gloves and dispose of them according to facility policy. Wash your hands. ☐ ☐ _____

18. Help the person back into a comfortable position, straighten the bottom linens, and draw the top linens over the person. Raise the head of the bed as the person requests. ☐ ☐ _____

19. Make sure the bed is lowered to its lowest position and the wheels are locked. If the side rails are in use, return them to the raised position. ☐ ☐ _____

20. Gather the soiled linens and place them in the linen hamper. Dispose of disposable items in a facility-approved waste container. ☐ ☐ _____

Finishing Up

21. Complete the "Finishing Up" steps. ☐ ☐ _____